QUALITY
HEALTH CARE

The Role of Continuing

Medical Education

Preparation of this volume was
assisted by a grant from The Robert
Wood Johnson Foundation,
Princeton, New Jersey. The opinions,
conclusions, or proposals in the
text are those of the authors and do
not necessarily represent the
views of The Robert Wood Johnson
Foundation.

Published in cooperation with

BOSTON UNIVERSITY
HEALTH POLICY INSTITUTE

QUALITY HEALTH CARE

The Role of Continuing Medical Education

Richard H. Egdahl, M.D., Ph.D.

and

Paul M. Gertman, M.D.

Editors

ASPEN SYSTEMS CORPORATION
GERMANTOWN, MARYLAND
1977

Library of Congress Catalog Card Number : 77-70434
ISBN: 0-912862-37-8

Printed in the United States of America.

1 2 3 4 5

Table of Contents

Contributors... xi
Preface... xv
Introduction... xvii

PART I —   CURRENT PROGRAMS IN
                CONTINUING MEDICAL EDUCATION...... 1

Chapter 1—   The Physician's Recognition Award:
                Relationship to Quality of Care 3
                PRA Purpose 3
                PRA Requirements...................... 4
                PRA and Quality of Care 5
                Critics of the PRA...................... 7
                Conclusion............................. 9

Chapter 2—   The Continuing Education Component
                of the Bi-Cycle Approach to Quality Assurance 11
                The Model 11
                Types of Change 13
                Health Care Problem Requiring Multiple and
                Specific Change Programs 16

Chapter 3—   Medical Practice Related to Continuing
                Education by Practice Profiling............ 19
                Method 20
                Results............................... 20
                Undeveloped Phase 22
                Discussion 23

Chapter 4—   The Physician Education Program and the Kaiser-
               Permanente System of Quality Assurance 29
               Introduction 29
               The Kaiser-Permanente Physician Education
               Program 30
               Comments and Observations 34

Chapter 5—   Do Self-Assessment Methods of Continuing
               Medical Education Affect Quality of Patient
               Care? 39
               The SESAP Programs 39
               Evaluation.............................. 43

PART II —   REQUIRED SYSTEMS OF CME PROGRAMS... 45

Chapter 6—   Reexamination/Recertification:
               Measurement of Professional Competence and
               Relation to Quality of Medical Care 47
               Evaluation Methodology 48
               Forces Influencing Recertification.......... 56
               Enabling Recertification 61

Chapter 7—   Recertification in Family Practice............ 63
               CME and Recertification: The Concept 63
               CME Documentation..................... 65
               Cognitive Examination.................... 66
               Office Record Review 66
               Possible Future Measures 67

Chapter 8—   Continuing Medical Education: The Role
               of the State and the Medical Society......... 69
               Malpractice and Licensure 70
               Public Policy Concerns 72
               Recommendations....................... 73
               Conclusion............................. 74

PART III —   EVALUATION OF CME PROGRAMS 77

Chapter 9—   The Impact of CME on the Quality of
               Care: What Are the Results?............... 79
               General Practitioners and CME............. 79
               Professionalizing CME.................... 82
               Other CME Studies....................... 85
               The Example of Florence Nightingale........ 89
               Conclusions 90

Chapter 10—   Evaluating the Evaluators of Continuing
     Medical Education Programs 93
     Traditional CME 94
     Recent Trends in CME 96

Chapter 11—   The Role of PSROs in Conducting and Evaluating
     Continuing Medical Education Programs. ... 101
     Quality Assurance. 101
     Education in Utilization Review 105
     The Role of PSRO in Consumer Education ... 105
     Evaluation of CME Programs. 106

PART IV —   FINANCIAL ASPECTS OF CME 107

Chapter 12—   Benefit-Cost Aspects of Continuing
     Medical Education 109
     Benefit-Cost Analysis: Some General
     Principles. 110
     Benefits of CME Programs. 112
     Costs of CME. 117
     Equity and Efficiency in CME 119
     Conclusion 126

Chapter 13—   The Internal Revenue Code and
     Continuing Medical Education. 131
     Tax Law. 131
     CME Expenses 133
     Policy Alternatives. 138

Chapter 14—   The Current Investment in Continuing
     Medical Education 143
     Physician Investment. 144
     Hospital Investment. 145
     Medical School Investment. 146
     Medical Association Investment 147
     Specialty Society Investment. 148
     Industry Investment. 148
     Government Investment 149
     Investment Summary. 151
     Return on Investment. 152
     Public Policy Issues 156

PART V —   POLICY ALTERNATIVES TO
              MANDATORY CME 161
Chapter 15—   Challenges to Continuing Medical Education . . 163
              Public Accountability and CME 164
              Where Current Programs Fail 165
              The Changes That Are Demanded 168

Chapter 16—   Can CME Be Made Part of a Medical
              Education Continuum? 173
              Is CME Effective? 174
              Can CME Improve Quality of Care? 175
              Improving Physician Habits 176
              Medical School Faculties and CME 177
              The Information Overload 178

Chapter 17—   Future Role of the Medical School, Community
              Hospital, and Medical Society in Continuing
              Medical Education 181
              Introduction 181
              Five Policy Recommendations 182
              Role of Medical Schools. 183
              Role of the Medical Societies 189
              Role of Hospitals 191
              Role of the Computer 191

Chapter 18—   Patient Education, Patient Compliance and the
              Continuing Education of Physicians 195
              How Are Physicians Informed about Drugs? . . 196
              Irrational Prescribing. 198
              Adverse Drug Reactions. 199
              Patient Attitudes and Actions— The Problem
              of Compliance 200
              The Role of the Physician and the Pharmacist
              in Patient Education 204

Chapter 19—   Health Education for Consumers: An
              Alternative to Continuing Education for
              Providers 211
              The Evidence. 212
              Another Look at the Evidence 215
              Conclusions 218

PART VI —   ISSUES FOR POLICY CONSIDERATION 221
Chapter 20— Policy Issues and Conclusions 223
             The Role of CME in Quality Assurance 225
             Form, Costs, and Evaluations of Mandatory
                 CME. 229
             The Future of CME. 232
PART VII—   Policy Recommendations of the Boston University
                 Health Policy Center 235
Chapter 21— Policy Recommendations. 237
Index 241

Editors

Paul M. Gertman, M.D.
CHIEF, HEALTH CARE
  RESEARCH SECTION
DIVISION OF MEDICINE
BOSTON UNIVERSITY SCHOOL
  OF MEDICINE

Richard H. Egdahl, M.D., Ph.D.
ACADEMIC VICE PRESIDENT FOR
  HEALTH AFFAIRS
BOSTON UNIVERSITY
DIRECTOR
BOSTON UNIVERSITY
  HEALTH POLICY INSTITUTE

Contributors

Daniel S. Bernstein, M.D.
ASSOCIATE DEAN FOR HOSPITAL
  AFFILIATIONS AND POSTGRADUATE
  EDUCATION
BOSTON UNIVERSITY
MEDICAL CENTER
BOSTON, MASSACHUSETTS

Clement R. Brown, Jr., M.D.
DIRECTOR, MEDICAL EDUCATION
SOUTH CHICAGO COMMUNITY
  HOSPITAL
CHICAGO, ILLINOIS

Frederic D. Berg, M.D.
DIRECTOR OF THE GRADUATE AND
  CONTINUING MEDICAL EVALUATION
  DEPARTMENT
NATIONAL BOARD OF MEDICAL
  EXAMINERS
PHILADELPHIA, PENNSYLVANIA

Rick J. Carlson, J.D.
HEALTH CONSULTANT
MILL VALLEY, CALIFORNIA

Robert A. Chase, M.D.
PRESIDENT, NATIONAL BOARD OF
  MEDICAL EXAMINERS
PHILADELPHIA, PENNSYLVANIA

John A.D. Cooper, M.D.
PRESIDENT, ASSOCIATION OF
  AMERICAN MEDICAL COLLEGES
WASHINGTON, D.C.

Gregory T. Halbert, J.D.
RESEARCH ASSOCIATE IN
  HEALTH LAW
DENVER, COLORADO

C. Rollins Hanlon, M.D.
DIRECTOR, AMERICAN COLLEGE
  OF SURGEONS
CHICAGO, ILLINOIS

Philip R. Lee, M.D.
DIRECTOR, UNIVERSITY OF
  CALIFORNIA HEALTH POLICY CENTER
SAN FRANCISCO, CALIFORNIA

Sol Levine, Ph.D.
PROFESSOR OF SOCIOLOGY AND
  COMMUNITY MEDICINE
BOSTON UNIVERSITY
BOSTON, MASSACHUSETTS

Philip R. Manning, M.D.
ASSOCIATE DEAN, UNIVERSITY OF
  SOUTHERN CALIFORNIA, SCHOOL
  OF MEDICINE,
POSTGRADUATE DIVISION
LOS ANGELES, CALIFORNIA

Elaine McDonald, B.A.
PROJECT SPECIALIST,
DEPARTMENT OF CONTINUING
MEDICAL EDUCATION
UNIVERSITY OF WISCONSIN
MADISON, WISCONSIN

George E. Miller, M.D.
DIRECTOR, CENTER FOR
EDUCATION DEVELOPMENT
UNIVERSITY OF ILLINOIS
MEDICAL CENTER
CHICAGO, ILLINOIS

Lewis A. Miller
PRESIDENT, MILLER AND
FINK CORPORATION
DARIEN, CONNECTICUT

Alan C. Monheit, Ph.D.
RESEARCH ASSOCIATE IN
HEALTH ECONOMICS
BOSTON UNIVERSITY HEALTH
POLICY INSTITUTE
BOSTON, MASSACHUSETTS

Alan R. Nelson, M.D.
INTERNIST
SALT LAKE CITY, UTAH

Osler Peterson, M.D.
PROFESSOR OF PREVENTIVE AND
SOCIAL MEDICINE
HARVARD SCHOOL OF PUBLIC HEALTH
BOSTON, MASSACHUSETTS

Leonard Rubin, M.D.
COORDINATOR OF EDUCATION
KAISER-PERMANENTE MEDICAL
GROUP OF NORTHERN
CALIFORNIA
OAKLAND, CALIFORNIA

C.H. William Ruhe, M.D.
SENIOR VICE PRESIDENT
AMERICAN MEDICAL ASSOCIATION
CHICAGO, ILLINOIS

Sigurd E. Sivertson, M.D.
ASSISTANT DEAN OF CONTINUING
MEDICAL EDUCATION
UNIVERSITY OF WISCONSIN
MADISON, WISCONSIN

J. Jerome Wildgen, M.D.
FAMILY PRACTITIONER
KALISPELL, MONTANA

Harold Zintel, M.D., F.A.C.S.
ASSISTANT DIRECTOR,
AMERICAN COLLEGE OF SURGEONS
CHICAGO, ILLINOIS

Other Conference Participants

Federal Invitees

Gregory J. Ahart, J.D.
DIRECTOR, MANPOWER AND
WELFARE DIVISION
GENERAL ACCOUNTING OFFICE
WASHINGTON, D.C.

Philip Caper, M.D.
PROFESSIONAL STAFF MEMBER,
LABOR AND PUBLIC WELFARE
SUBCOMMITTEE ON HEALTH
WASHINGTON, D.C.

James Dickson, III, M.D.
DEPUTY ASSISTANT SECRETARY
FOR HEALTH
DEPARTMENT OF HEALTH,
EDUCATION, AND WELFARE
WASHINGTON, D.C.

Kenneth M. Endicott, M.D.
ADMINISTRATOR, HEALTH RESOURCES
ADMINISTRATION
DEPARTMENT OF HEALTH,
EDUCATION, AND WELFARE
ROCKVILLE, MARYLAND

Michael J. Goran, M.D.
DIRECTOR, BUREAU OF QUALITY
ASSURANCE, HEALTH SERVICES
ADMINISTRATION
DEPARTMENT OF HEALTH,
EDUCATION, AND WELFARE
ROCKVILLE, MARYLAND

Stanley Wallack
CHIEF OF HEALTH AND VETERANS
AFFAIRS, CONGRESSIONAL
BUDGET OFFICE
HUMAN RESOURCES DIVISION
WASHINGTON, D.C.

Other Invitees

Robert H. Barnes, M.D.
DIRECTOR, HEALTH CARE
REVIEW CENTER
SEATTLE, WASHINGTON

Jonathan Fielding, M.D.
COMMISSIONER OF PUBLIC HEALTH
COMMONWEALTH OF MASSACHUSETTS
BOSTON, MASSACHUSETTS

Ruby P. Hearn, Ph.D.
PROGRAM OFFICER, ROBERT
WOOD JOHNSON FOUNDATION
PRINCETON, NEW JERSEY

Verne Horn
DIRECTOR, CENTER FOR
HEALTH POLICY
GEORGETOWN UNIVERSITY
WASHINGTON, D.C.

William D. Mayer, M.D.
DIRECTOR, HEALTH SERVICES
RESEARCH AND DEVELOPMENT
CENTER
UNIVERSITY OF MISSOURI
COLUMBIA, MISSOURI

Judith Miller
HEALTH STAFF SEMINAR
GEORGE WASHINGTON UNIVERSITY
WASHINGTON, D.C.

John Moses, M.D.
SECRETARY, MICHIGAN MEDICAL
PRACTICE BOARD
DIRECTOR OF MEDICAL EDUCATION
MT. CARMEL MERCY HOSPITAL
AND MEDICAL CENTER
DETROIT, MICHIGAN

John I. Sandson, M.D.
DEAN, BOSTON UNIVERSITY
SCHOOL OF MEDICINE
BOSTON, MASSACHUSETTS

Frederick Stone, Ph.D.
DEPUTY DIRECTOR, BOSTON
UNIVERSITY MEDICAL CENTER
BOSTON, MASSACHUSETTS

Claude Welch, M.D.
CHAIRMAN, BOARD OF REGISTRATION
AND DISCIPLINE IN MEDICINE
COMMONWEALTH OF
MASSACHUSETTS
SENIOR CONSULTANT IN SURGERY
MASSACHUSETTS GENERAL
HOSPITAL
BOSTON, MASSACHUSETTS

Edward Roberts, Ph.D.
SARNOFF PROFESSOR
SLOAN SCHOOL, MASSACHUSETTS
INSTITUTE OF TECHNOLOGY
CAMBRIDGE, MASSACHUSETTS

Boston University Health Policy Institute Staff

Director:

Richard H. Egdahl, M.D., Ph.D.
ACADEMIC VICE-PRESIDENT FOR
HEALTH AFFAIRS,
BOSTON UNIVERSITY
DIRECTOR, BOSTON UNIVERSITY
MEDICAL CENTER

Senior Advisers:

George J. Annas, J.D., M.P.H.
DIRECTOR, BOSTON
UNIVERSITY CENTER FOR LAW AND
HEALTH SCIENCES

Paul M. Gertman, M.D.
DIRECTOR, HEALTH SERVICES
RESEARCH AND DEVELOPMENT
BOSTON UNIVERSITY MEDICAL
CENTER

Sol Levine, Ph.D.
PROFESSOR OF SOCIOLOGY AND
COMMUNITY MEDICINE, UNIVERSITY
PROFESSOR
BOSTON UNIVERSITY

Research Associates:

John Blum, J.D., M.P.H.
RESEARCH ASSOCIATE IN
HEALTH LAW

Donald R. Giller, M.S.
RESEARCH ASSOCIATE IN
HEALTH COMMUNICATIONS

Alan Monheit, Ph.D.
RESEARCH ASSOCIATE IN
HEALTH ECONOMICS

Cynthia H. Taft, B.A.
RESEARCH ASSOCIATE IN
HEALTH PLANNING

Kenneth J. Linde, M.P.H.
SENIOR HEALTH POLICY ANALYST

Regina A. Robbins, B.A.
ADMINISTRATIVE ASSISTANT

Pamela A. Hull
SECRETARY

Preface

This volume of nineteen essays examining the hows, whys, and wherefores of the link between continuing medical education and quality health care arose out of a conference in Boston in June 1976. The meeting was the second in a series of semiannual conferences conducted by the Boston University Program on Public Policy for Quality Health Care, under a grant from The Robert Wood Johnson Foundation of Princeton, New Jersey. The goal of the meetings was to provide a forum for cogent, in-depth discussion by individuals from the public and private sectors who have major involvement in policy issues affecting the quality of health care. The topic of this second conference was selected because of the virtual flood of recent legislative and regulatory activities in the area of continuing medical education, as well as efforts in recertification and relicensure by professional organizations.

The forty-two individuals who participated in the June seminar represented a wide range of viewpoints on continuing medical education and its link to quality health care. To provide the participants with a common ground for discussion and debate, nineteen background papers were prepared under the aegis of the Program on Public Policy for Quality Health Care and distributed in advance of the meeting; these papers compose the core of this volume. Prepared by acknowledged authorities on each respective topic, the papers represent a valuable compendium of current thought about the broad field of continuing medical education and quality health care.

The June meeting was devoted to open discussion aimed at clarifying differences of opinion and exposing participants to meaningful debate on the policy alternatives. The recommendations that flowed from the conference discussions were refined by the staff and published in November 1976 as *Continuing Medical Education and Quality*

Health Care: What is the Link? (Copies can be obtained from the Boston University Health Policy Institute, 53 Bay State Road, Boston, Massachusetts 02115.) That monograph contains a discussion of policy alternatives in the field of continuing medical education, as well as a summary of the conference discussions and participants' comments. The summary, excerpted comments, and policy recommendations are contained at the end of this volume.

The Program on Public Policy for Quality Health Care is a part of the Boston University Health Policy Center. Future meetings being planned will examine technology in medicine and quality of care in corporate health systems. It is our hope that these meetings, background papers, and policy monographs will represent an important contribution toward the improvement of quality and the delivery of health services.

RICHARD H. EGDAHL, M.D., Ph.D.
Boston
March 1977

Introduction

Although continuing education for physicians past their formal medical school and specialty training is a well-enshrined tradition of the profession, it has long been a low priority—even "backwater"—public policy issue for both the profession and for government. In fact, for many physicians, continuing medical education (CME) activities have often been regarded as a means of vacationing or participating in leisure activities while obtaining sizable tax deductions. In the last several years, however, there has been a virtual explosion of interest and activitiy in CME. After a decade of only modest increases, the number of CME courses offered has grown almost 50 percent a year for the last two years; fourteen state medical societies in recent years have set requirements for CME as a condition of membership; and ten states now directly require a physician to enroll in a specified amount of CME courses a year (or allow their licensing boards to establish such requirements) as a condition to maintain a physician's license to practice medicine. Almost all these new efforts are being carried out in the name of ensuring physician competence, thereby assuring the public of quality medical care.

With this activity there has come confusion, acrimony, and concern over definitions of continuing medical education; content of educational activities; the need for mandatory, as opposed to voluntary, programs; the relationship of education to malpractice issues; and the effectiveness of CME in improving the competence of physicians and/or the health of the public. In particular, as the movement for mandatory CME as a condition of licensure or certification has spread, CME has moved from a peripheral issue to a topic of major importance for state government and physicians in those states.

In furtherance of its responsibility to identify issues of national importance, to delineate the specifics of such issues, and to clarify options and/or make recommendations for government, the Boston University Health Policy Institute convened a conference of national experts to discuss "the relationship of continuing medical education to the quality of medical care." To stimulate discussion and focus on problem areas, it was decided to request that nineteen of the conference participants prepare in advance brief background essays that would review a variety of issues about CME and the quality of medical care. This book is a collection of those background papers and of Boston University's synthesis of issues and recommendations emanating from the conference, which was held in June 1976.

The background papers are related to the five topic areas that the conference was expected to deal with: current voluntary programs in CME; mandated or required systems of CME; evaluation of CME programs; financial aspects of CME; and policy issues for consideration by the conference participants. Although each of the essays stands in its own right, it is worth briefly reviewing for the reader the nature of the papers, the rationale for the five general topics, and how each of the papers related to the topics. It should be kept in mind that the papers were written as background to a conference, not as scholarly works; and they are being published as part of the Boston University program's effort to make information from its public policy activities broadly available.

The first background topic (and the first part of this volume) was intended to present brief reviews of examples of different aspects of and approaches to *voluntary* efforts in continuing medical education. The first paper, by C.H. William Ruhe of the American Medical Association, succinctly summarizes the intent, content and expected accomplishment of the AMA's Physician's Recognition Award program. This award (which requires that a physician undertake 150 hours of a mix of formal and informal CME activities over a three-year period) represents an articulation of a belief that a minimum amount of continued learning is essential to the maintenance of an acceptable level of competence by physicians. It emphasizes the concept of a "floor," rather than supporting any particular education approach. The second paper, by Clement R. Brown, Jr., a leader in hospital-based medical audit work, takes the opposite tack of emphasizing approach over requirements. It presents an updated version of the continuing education component of Brown's now-famous "Bi-Cycle" approach to quality assurance, which combines problem identification through medical audit with a set of change activities designed to correct identified problems. It is a particularly important approach because it has, with little modification, been adopted as the basic program of quality assurance under the federal Professional Standards Review Organization (PSRO) program. Brown carefully notes that many problems of assuring quality go beyond transferring information to physicians. Often that requires confronting the difficult area of behavioral and attitudinal changes by patients and physicians, as well as changes in health care system organization and resources.

Sigurd E. Silvertson, assistant dean of the University of Wisconsin College of Medicine, and his associate, Elaine McDonald, describe a relatively new and exciting approach to improving quality of care that they and their colleagues at the University of Wisconsin have been developing in recent years. In contrast to the hospital-based orientation of Brown, Sivertson and his colleagues have attempted to build a relationship directly between office-based general practitioners and the state university medical center. They do this through the development of individual practice profiles that contrast the physician's actual practice against self-assessment exams; these profiles are then used to feed back individually tailored recommendations for improving competence through continuing education. Another model of an areawide system for continuing medical education is presented in Leonard Rubin's description of the Kaiser-Permanente system of quality assurance. Kaiser's coherent administration and organization, combined with local flexibility in approach, will be of interest to many planners of regionalized systems. Harold A. Zintel and C. Rollins Hanlon, of the American College of Surgeons, argue the case for the use of the computerized self-assessment examination as a mainstay of future CME activities and for its superiority over traditional teaching modalities, such as lectures. Although the specific activities discussed in each of these five papers are not mutually exclusive, they represent a considerable variation in emphasis on the types of problems that exist in assuring quality and maintaining physician competence and on the different approaches to attacking such problems.

Part II deals with a major force for continuing education in recent years—the trend toward concepts of periodic recertification and relicensure, based not only on mandatory participation in continuing education but also on actual reexamination. The key organizational actors in this area have been predominantly the medical specialty boards, whose history and current activities with respect to reexamination and recertification requirements are reviewed by Robert A. Chase and Frederick D. Burg, of the National Board of Medical Examiners. They also present a succinct synthesis of the forces driving toward recertification by the specialty boards, the forces acting as a restraining influence, and the actions that various private and public agencies might take to enhance the drive toward comprehensive specialty recertification programs. The "pace-setter" in the recertification field has been the American Board of Family Practice, whose program of mandatory CME hours, licensure checks, office record reviews, and reexaminations is presented by J. Jerome Wildgen, a Montana family practitioner. The results of this program, which will give its first reexaminations in 1977, will be closely watched throughout the nation. The third paper on the topic of mandatory programs deals with the subject of relicensure of physicians by state governments. Daniel S. Bernstein, associate dean of Boston University School of Medicine, not only reviews the current "score card" on state requirements for mandatory CME and relicensure but also criticizes the lack of substantive focus of such regulations and urges the development of specific mechanisms for integrating PSRO activities and findings with the relicensure and disciplinary powers of state boards.

The authors of Part III were asked to address themselves specifically to evaluating the data on whether continuing medical education improves physician competence and the quality of patient care. Osler Peterson of the Harvard Medical School examines a variety of studies, including some unpublished data from his famous study of North Carolina practitioners in the 1950s and newer studies contrasting clinical decisions by doctors and computers. He also makes the important point that evaluations of CME have a difficult methodologic problem in that effects of education are often hard to differentiate from effects of organization. The importance of organizational settings and the incentives and sanctions that they have available to influence the quality of medical care are also noted in the paper by Sol Levine, a Boston University medical sociologist. After reviewing the evidence from the small number of evaluation studies which generally show that CME has no effect on the quality of care, Levine points out that the CME participated in by physicians has usually been of such minimal amount that to use this as an input variable in evaluating CME's ability to change quality of medical care is not a fair test. Further, Levine is highly critical both of the general lack of evaluation of CME programs and the absence of scientific rigor in what little evaluation has been conducted. The final background paper on evaluation, by Alan R. Nelson, deals with the role of PSROs. Nelson is a member of the National Professional Standards Review Council, and based on the pioneering experiences of the Utah Professional Review Organization, he concludes that the types of problems found through medical audit do not readily lend themselves to correction through formalized continuing medical education—nor does simple identification of such problems lead to changes in physician behavior. This experience, if found elsewhere, will be a severe disappointment to many within both the medical community and government agencies who have hoped to link PSRO findings closely with formal CME activities.

Part IV deals with a topic that has received only superficial consideration in the past—the financial aspects of CME activities. To start this section, Alan C. Monheit, a health economist at Boston University, attempts to delineate for the first time the theoretical issues involved in developing a cost-benefit calculation for evaluating continuing medical education programs. Monheit points out the complex factors, such as potential reduction in services to patients by time spent on CME, new techniques learned that might increase a physician's income, the diminishing period of potential return on CME as a physician ages, and many others, factors that must be considered in developing a cost-benefit analysis. Monheit's personal doubt is that the benefit-cost ratio for traditional CME activities would exceed unity if the data were available to do such a calculation. Gregory T. Halbert, a health attorney, points out in his chapter that one of the major financial forces stimulating CME activities is the availability of income tax deduction benefits to physicians, and he carefully reviews how such deductions are determined. Lewis A. Miller, a publisher and CME consultant, attempts to develop an actual estimate of the current expenditures being made by physicians, medical schools, government agencies, the pharmaceutical industry, hospitals, medical societies, and others on continuing medical education. He estimates a direct cost of $400 million, plus another $1.4 billion in income loss to physicians because of participation in CME. However, he notes that it is almost impossible to assess the return of this investment, since benefits sought from CME are not easily monetized.

The focus of the conference was the definition of the policy issues, and the chapters in Part V served as useful starting points for the expert debate. George E. Miller, a leading expert on medical education evaluation, challenges many of the current policies and directions of CME efforts, which he believes are both simplistic in nature and inadequate to improve the quality of medical care. Though he believes there are no simple answers or solutions, Miller advocates development of lifetime programs of CME for physicians and wants to see the authority for CME taken away from existing power groups and placed in the hands of special regional consortia. The president of the Association of American Medical Colleges, John A.D. Cooper, notes that one national commission after another has recommended that medical schools assume the key institutional responsibility for developing continuing medical education programs, but they have not done so. He cites as some of the reasons for this the increased tightening of funds, responsibilities for larger undergraduate classes, lack of status for faculty members doing CME, and increasing doubts about whether traditional forms of CME are useful. Cooper believes that medical schools can make a major contribution by training medical students— and thus future physicians—to develop skills of self-criticism and care assessment and to possess independent learning traits so they will be better prepared for a lifetime of continuing education. In partial contrast to Cooper and in virtual opposition to Miller, Philip R. Manning of the University of Southern California argues in his paper that the medical schools should, in fact, assume the formal lead responsibility for CME activities. He supports the notion that multiple organizations currently involved in hospitals, PSROs, specialty boards, medical schools, etc., each continue their activities and loosely coordinate them through the Liaison Committee on Continuing Medical Education.

Philip R. Lee, professor of social medicine at the University of California (and a former assistant secretary for health) approaches the quality assurance/continuing education interface from a different point of view. He believes that in one of the major health care problem areas—drug prescribing, compliance, and side effects—the most effective way to improve health status might be better education of the patient, rather than the physician. He points out that much of what is wrong in this area may be due to the way physicians have been educated by drug detail men (also noting the control of the drug industry over much of the medical educational media). Lee suggests expansion of the concept of package inserts for patients and a greater role for pharmacists in patient education when physicians cannot or will not take the time to provide this service. The case for a national program of consumer health education—as a public policy alternative to expanded physician continuing education—is made even more broadly and pungently by Rick J. Carlson, a well-known critic of the current American medical system. Carlson believes that mass consumer health education could represent a revolutionary turning point in improving the health status of the American people.

Finally, the last part of this volume presents the views of the staff of the Boston University Health Policy Institute on the relationship of continuing medical education to the quality of medical care and the comments made by conference participants on some facets of this linkage. It further contains the staff's recommendations for actions the

State and Federal governments might take to further continuing medical education activities.

It is hoped that this collection of background essays will give the reader concerned with continuing medical education and public policy a better understanding of the various possible programs and their potential effects on improving the health of the American people.

PAUL M. GERTMAN, M.D.
Boston
March 1977

Part I

Current Programs in Continuing Medical Education

Chapter 1
The Physician's Recognition Award: Relationship to Quality of Care

C. H. William Ruhe

The acknowledged goal of all continuing medical education is improved quality of patient care. Whether that goal is achieved depends on a number of factors, only one of which is the quality of education provided. Timeliness, relevance, practicability, and applicability are also factors of great importance, as are the motivation and dedication of the learners.

PRA PURPOSE

It is these latter factors which the Physician's Recognition Award (PRA) attempts to address. The PRA was established by action of the American Medical Association (AMA) House of Delegates in 1968 after several years of consideration and development of the idea by AMA staff and an Advisory Committee of the AMA Board of Trustees on Continuing Medical Education. The major purposes were "to provide recognition for the many thousands of physicians who regularly participate in continuing medical education" and "to encourage each physician to keep up-to-date and to improve his knowledge and judgment by continuing medical education."

The philosophy was simple: it was based on the assumption that continuing medical education is desirable, that every physician should participate in it, and that physicians are more likely to do so if they receive some recognition for it. These principles were elaborated in a formal report adopted by the AMA's House of Delegates in 1973, "A Policy Statement on Continuing Medical Education." A portion of this statement reads as follows:

The American Medical Association believes strongly that regular participation in continuing medical education is

3

essential to the maintenance of professional competence. The AMA believes that every member of the Association and every other physician should plan and engage voluntarily in a regular program of continuing education designed to maintain his personal professional competence.

The AMA Physician's Recognition Award has been established as a means of recognizing physicians who participate in a stated amount of continuing education on a regular basis. The standards for the Award represent an expression of an acceptable level of involvement in continuing medical education for every physician. The American Medical Association urges every physician to meet or exceed the standards of the Physician's Recognition Award in his personal program of continuing medical education.

PRA REQUIREMENTS

To obtain the Physician's Recognition Award, a physician must complete 150 credit hours of continuing medical education (CME) within a three-year period. Of these, at least sixty hours must be in Category 1 (it is possible for all 150 to be in Category 1). There are five other categories in which credit may be earned, but the amount of credit applicable toward the 150 hours is limited for each of the other categories, as follows:

Category	Description	Credit Hour Limit
1.	CME activities with accredited sponsorship	No limit
2.	CME activities with nonaccredited sponsorship	45 hours
3.	Medical teaching	45 hours
4.	Papers, publications, books, exhibits	40 hours
5.	Nonsupervised individual CME	45 hours
6.	Other meritorious learning experiences	45 hours

The requirement that there be at least sixty hours in Category 1 with no limit on the total that may be credited from this category is an attempt to assure that a significant part of the CME activities will be taken in programs offered by accredited institutions. This ties the recognition of the individual to the system for accreditation of the institution or organization, as is the case for other levels of medical education. Although there is no guarantee that the educational offering of the accredited institution will meet the needs of the physician-learner, there is some assurance that it is a planned program, with defined objectives, attempting to cover a circumscribed body of information or set of skills, and that the institution or organization that presents it is capable of providing education of acceptable quality.

The other categories available for credit are offered because there is general agreement that physicians can learn in a variety of ways and that no single educational experience is necessarily the best for all physicians. Category 2 provides credit for attendance at scientific meetings or other continuing education activities of institutions that have not been accredited, acknowledging that there can be meritorious programs under nonaccredited auspices. Category 3 provides credit for the medical teacher, respecting the fact that every teacher must learn in preparation for teaching. It does not, however, relieve the teacher of the responsibility for furthering his own education through regular participation in formal educational programs. Category 4 acknowledges the learning experience from the preparation of a scientific paper for presentation before a medical society, or for publication in a scientific journal, from writing a book, or from preparing a scientific exhibit. Category 5 permits the individual who prefers to learn by reading or self-study to obtain some credit for doing so, even though it is done in an unsupervised fashion. Category 6 is made available to permit the applicant to request credit for some unusual individualized type of learning experience. Specific questions must be answered concerning the nature of the experience, the technique used, and the supervision provided before such credit is allowable.

PRA AND QUALITY OF CARE

What does all this have to do with quality of care? Does the PRA have any direct relevance to quality of care? Can it be shown that the physician who earns the PRA provides better quality of care than the physician who does not? Can it be shown that the physician who earns the PRA provides better care as a result of having gone through the procedures to earn the PRA? The answers to these questions must be essentially negative if direct documentation of improved quality of care is required for a positive response.

The relationship is—and probably always will be—indirect, since there are many steps between participation in an educational program and improved performance in caring for patients. Knowledge and performance are not the same thing: there are many reasons why a person performs in a certain way in a given setting, and his level of knowledge is only one of these. Similarly, it is important to remember that knowledge is not necessarily the same thing as education, or at least not formal education.

The argument that participation in the PRA will lead to improved patient care is the same argument that one might use in favor of any kind of formal education. There is no direct proof that attendance at medical school and obtaining the M.D. degree makes an individual a better physician, or that participation in residency training makes an individual a better physician, or that specialty board certification in itself assures that an individual is a more competent physician. In each case the evidence is indirect, but one usually does not question the need for such formal education. Only continuing medical education seems to need to prove itself by providing direct documentation of improved quality of care.

It is frequently difficult to provide such documentation for any individual CME activity. The main problem is that the amount of learning that results from an individual continuing education course is but a small part of his total body of knowledge and experience. It is only when the individual course is aimed at a specific new skill or technique, or when it concerns a new piece of information that will be directly useful, that we can demonstrate a measurable change in the physician's behavior.

Nevertheless, there are certain principles that seem to support the belief that continuing education is valuable and that it has an influence on quality of care. First, it is impossible to use knowledge or a skill that one does not have. The person with that knowledge or skill might not always use it efficiently or meritoriously in practice, but the person without it has no opportunity at all.

The second principle is that the level of information retained decreases continuously if it is not refreshed or used regularly. One of the most important reasons for participating in CME is to renew knowledge gained at an earlier period. The rainfall that keeps the level of a pond constant might be likened to individual continuing education programs. It would be difficult to show a specific effect from an individual drop of rain or even from a brief shower. Yet without that periodic addition, evaporation would surely lower the level.

The third important principle is that there is considerable value in peer pressure, both in motivation to learn and in quality of performance. Regular participation in continuing education in concert with other physicians is unquestionably beneficial to the individual physician. Most physicians have a considerable amount of professional pride; they have come up through a competitive system requiring them to demonstrate their qualifications at various points along the way. The discipline of continuing medical education refurbishes professional pride and exposes the individual physician to peer pressure which, in turn, encourages him or her to learn and perform better.

CRITICS OF THE PRA

There are those who maintain that there is little value in a "brownie point" system that allows physicians credit for individual courses taken or for participation in other types of learning experiences. Usually those who take this position argue that only direct audit of a physician's performance, at either the process or the outcome level, bears any significant relationship to continued competence. Audit procedures are unquestionably meritorious, but they also have their drawbacks. For one thing, they are always retrospective rather than prospective; and, for another, they can only measure procedures or outcomes against standards that have been developed by peer group identification. They do not have any relation to the total body of knowledge or the total body of information possessed by individuals, and they are useful only when applied to specific educational programs which have direct relevance to an easily identified and measured knowledge or skill.

Evaluation can be carried out in a variety of ways at a variety of levels, from counting registrations at an individual course offering to complex socio-cultural-economic studies that attempt to determine whether the public has better health and is in a better state of happiness and well being. Figure 1-1 shows some of the varying measures that might be made on an increasingly complex scale of values. At the moment, the Physician's Recognition Award falls rather low on the scale since it attempts only to identify participation in continuing medical education. However, since the PRA is tied to accreditation of institutions and organizations offering continuing education, it has a built-in, gradually increasing set of standards. This results from the requirement that Category 1 credit allowances are tied to an institution's demonstration of defined objectives and its formal evaluation of programs identified as being of Category 1 quality. As institutions are subjected to continuing review in the accreditation cycle, more will be required of them toward demonstrating that they have met these standards. Accordingly, Category 1 will become more significant in time.

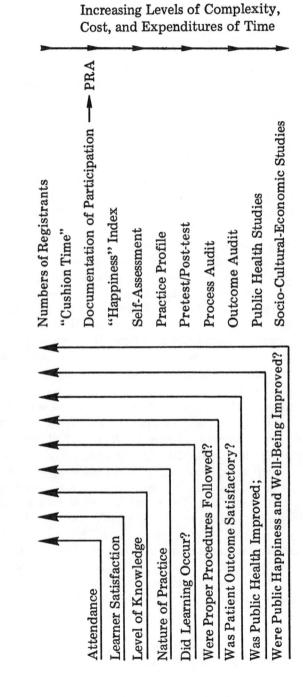

Figure 1-1
EVALUATION OF CONTINUING MEDICAL EDUCATION

CONCLUSION

For the present, as is noted in the beginning of this chapter, the PRA is based on certain assumptions: that continuing medical education is desirable, that every physician should participate in it, and that physicians are more likely to do so if they receive some recognition. In addition, the PRA serves as a standard for state boards of medical examiners, state medical associations, specialty societies, and others that are likely to institute formal CME requirements for membership or licensure. As such, the PRA constitutes a valuable national resource.

No one could argue that the PRA should substitute for self-assessment, peer review, medical audit, practice profiles, or any other types of evaluation of physician performance. At this point in the evolution of CME, however, the PRA serves as a valuable incentive to physicians to engage in continuing education, as well as a standard method of recognition for such participation.

Chapter 2
The Continuing Education Component of the Bi-Cycle Approach to Quality Assurance

Clement R. Brown, Jr.

THE MODEL

The "Bi-Cycle" Model (Figure 2-1) has provided the basis for the design of systems to assure the quality of patient and health care.[1,2] The model includes an outer *patient and health care cycle* and an inner *change or education cycle*. In this latest version of the model the inner cycle will be called the change cycle rather than the education cycle because most health professionals tend to think of education in a much more restricted sense than we have ever intended. Steps 10 through 12 on the change cycle represent the assurance component of the quality assurance system, as differentiated from the prior steps on the patient and health care cycle, which represent the assessment component of the quality assurance system. Included in the prior steps of the Bi-Cycle Model is a medical audit subsystem that identifies those health system, health professional, and patient changes that must occur to improve health and health care.

Steps 10 through 12 provide the program to achieve change, where necessary, to improve health care. When behavioral change of the health professional is required, the change program should be an educational program. However, the change needed to improve health care might not rest with individual health professional behavior; it may be a health care resource change involving equipment, space or personnel, or a change in the administrative or organizational structure of the health care delivery system; or in its governance.

Often, too, patient behavioral change is required to achieve improved health care. An effective quality assurance program requires that the patient assume the ultimate responsibility for his or her health and health care. Thus, the first step in this latest version of the

Figure 2-1

THE QUALITY ASSURANCE SYSTEM

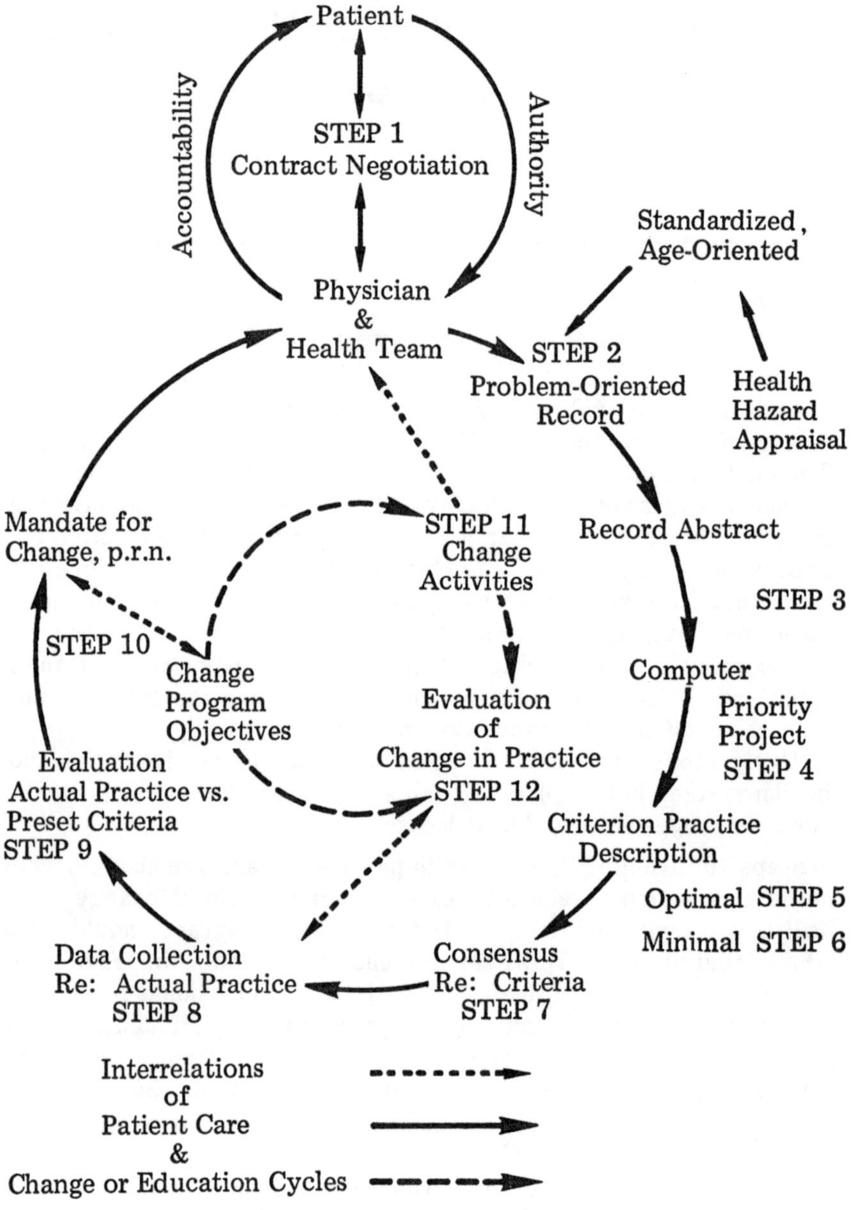

Patient

Accountability

Authority

STEP 1
Contract Negotiation

Standardized,
Age-Oriented

Physician
&
Health Team

STEP 2
Problem-Oriented
Record

Health
Hazard
Appraisal

Mandate for
Change, p.r.n.

STEP 11
Change
Activities

Record Abstract

STEP 3

STEP 10

Change
Program
Objectives

Evaluation
of
Change in Practice
STEP 12

Computer

Priority
Project
STEP 4

Evaluation
Actual Practice vs.
Preset Criteria
STEP 9

Criterion Practice
Description

Optimal STEP 5

Minimal STEP 6

Data Collection
Re: Actual Practice
STEP 8

Consensus
Re: Criteria
STEP 7

Interrelations
of
Patient Care
&
Change or Education Cycles

Source: Clement R. Brown, Jr., M.D. "Bi-Cycle Concept," 1976

Bi-Cycle Model is the development of a contract in which the patient agrees to accept this responsibility.

The change program objectives defined in Step 10 in the change cycle are derived from the assessment made in Step 9, the final health care assessment step. When actual performance is compared with criterion performance in Step 9 and deficiencies are identified, one need ask only: "Who must do what to move care from where we found it to where we have set our criteria?" These corrective behaviors in the health system, health professional, or patient become the objectives for the change or education program.

In Step 11, the programs for implementing and managing change are developed, and the specific activities to achieve change are carried out. In the experience in working with over 400 hospital groups during the past five years, this is the step in which it has been most difficult to achieve success, the step where most quality assurance programs grind to a halt. And, if "change, where necessary, to improve care" is the bottom line of a quality assurance program, lack of success in this step represents program failure.

Probably the most frequent cause for program failure in Step 11, although others will be reviewed momentarily, is the tendency of the managers of change to plan a change program that involves the health professional in learning something the change program director presumes the health professional does not know. Indeed, most change or corrective action programs take the form of educational programs that provide knowledge and perform information transfer. A true lack of knowledge on the part of the health professional is, however, a relatively infrequent cause of inferior patient care. If the review system manager and all participants in the health care system, including each patient, take a broader view of potential changes that must be made to improve the quality of health and health care, more effective "quality assurance" will result.

TYPES OF CHANGE

The types of change most frequently required to improve the quality of health and health care seem to fall into four groups:

1. patient behavior change,
2. health professional behavior change,
3. health care system change, and
4. health care resource change.

Patient Behavior Change

Probably the greatest potential for improved health maintenance lies in a change in the general life style or specific behaviors of the patients. It seems essential that patients assume the ultimate responsibility for these changes. Thus, the first step in the Bi-Cycle Model is the development of a contract between the patient and the health professional(s) in which the patient assumes this responsibility.

It then becomes the role of the health professional to provide the patient with data enabling the patient to make informed decisions with respect to activities that influence his or her health. For example, the greatest reduction in risk of death and disability by a patient who is a white male between the ages of 5 and 35 can be achieved by the regular use of seat belts. This information should be shared with all patients in this group.

As another example, although arterioslerotic heart disease does not become the top cause of death among white males until age 35, it is imperative to provide this cohort at an early age with the data on exercise, body weight, cigarette smoking, diet, and hypertension from which such patients can make informed decisions concerning the modification of any or all these risk factors. It might be most helpful among teenage males to help them achieve skills to cope with the peer pressure regarding cigarette smoking. It might not be helpful at all to warn them that the consequence of their starting to smoke cigarettes at age 14 is an increased risk of coronary artery disease at age 35, since teenagers live so much for the present. The health professional might instead relate their actual or potential cigarette smoking to a reduction in present capacity for long distance running, if they are participating in an active sports program.

Health Professional Behavior Change

Our behavior as health professionals in delivering health care can influence the health care outcomes of our patients, although probably not as much as we tend to think. Our behavior in delivering health care is influenced by knowledge, our skills (both mental and psychomotor), our attitudes, and the health care system in which we operate — as well as by the behavior of our patients.

Study of the use of antibiotics by the members of the medical department of Chestnut Hill Hospital in Pennsylvania revealed that in only 30 percent of instances of antibiotic use was the drug necessary and used appropriately. It might have been presumed that the physicians lacked knowledge of appropriate antibiotic usage, but this presumption was tested by administering a knowledge and problem-solving exam to the physicians. The average score on the test was 70 percent, revealing some knowledge and problem-solving deficit—but also revealing a knowledge and problem-solving level twice the practice level. It would not have been enough to develop a program that provided for information transfer and acquisition of better problem-solving skills with reference to antibiotic usage, although the learning experiences constructed did provide for such opportunities. It was also found that a number of physicians were afraid to withhold antibiotics when presented with a sick patient and an elevated temperature. The required attitudinal change was achieved through small group discussions in which physicians were able to value more highly the withholding of antibiotics until definitive data were obtained substantiating their use. This seems to point up the major deficiency of CME programs: they provide only for information transfer and do not provide opportunities for practicing problem-solving or achieving attitudinal change.

A review of the cardiopulmonary resuscitation (CPR) procedure in a hospital revealed that antiarrhythmic drug usage was delayed. Delay was due not to lack of knowledge of appropriate drug usage, but to lack of skill in venipuncture. It was necessary to provide opportunities to acquire the skill of venipuncture under the adverse conditions of cardiopulmonary resuscitation. A lecture about CPR, even with the assistance of film or videotape, would not have provided acquisition of the requisite skill. CME activities, therefore, must do more than just provide information.

Health Care System Change

During the course of the educational program described above to improve antibiotic usage, it became quite apparent that, while most physicians had responded on the examination that they would culture the throat of a patient with pharyngitis before prescribing an antibiotic, they were not so practicing because they lacked culture media and incubators in their office. An organizational or system change corrected this deficit. The hospital laboratory began a service of collecting throat cultures and other materials from physicians' offices for daily analysis.

In one hospital under study, physicians were responding inappropriately to laboratory data on urine cultures by ignoring high colony counts. The basis for this inappropriate response was found to be lack of trust in the laboratory reports: physicians knew that many urine cultures were delayed in reaching the laboratory, with resultant bacterial growth in the specimen bottle. Resolution of the problem was achieved when physicians were assured that samples for culture were refrigerated promptly on the ward to offset any delay in pick-up by the laboratory staff.

Health Care Resource Change

The members of the surgical department of a hospital agreed that most patients undergoing an elective cholecystectomy should have an operative cholangiogram. A review of actual practice revealed that less than half such patients had an operative cholangiogram because at the time the procedure should have been performed the only x-ray equipment available in surgery was in use elsewhere, most often for hip nailing. Resolution of this problem occurred with the purchase of additional x-ray equipment.

A high rate of postoperative infection was determined to be associated with surgery in one operating room. The hospital engineer determined that the air flow in the duct that was supposedly exhausting the room air was moving in the wrong direction. Correction of duct flow returned the postoperative infection rate to an acceptable level.

These are but two examples of the benefits of a resource change. Another that might be considered: high rates of nosocomial infection in a hospital can often be reduced by the addition of a nurse epidemologist to the staff. And on a less technical level: an inadequate data base on patients in an ambulatory setting can often be corrected by the use of allied health patient data gatherers. Each health care facility must seek solutions in its own situational experience.

HEALTH CARE PROBLEM REQUIRING MULTIPLE AND SPECIFIC CHANGE PROGRAMS

Improvement in the number of pelvic and Pap examinations done on hospitalized patients required a number of different and specific change programs in a hospital:

- One group of physicians placed little value on periodic pelvic and Pap exams for cervical and uterine malignancy. Small group discussions were used to achieve attitudinal change in this group.

- A second group of physicians valued the examinations but did not know how to perform them. This group was given the opportunity to practice performing pelvic and Pap exams under observation until they gave evidence of having acquired the necessary skill.
- A third group of physicians did not know how to perform the exam but chose not to learn this skill. This group agreed to have the procedure performed by allied health professionals or by other physicians, after being given assurance that they would retain the patients for the remainder of care.

The above discussion has centered on the second step on the inner change or education cycle of the Bi-Cycle Model (Figure 2-1). Presented here were some specific examples of changes required to improve the quality of health and health care for each of four types of change: patient behavior change, health professional behavior change, health care system change, and health care resource change. We have seen that, while the change program to achieve improved health and patient care might be a standard health professional education program, more often it is not, since the standard CME program is constructed to achieve only information transfer. Such programs are directed at providing knowledge, and lack of knowledge seldom seems to be the cause of health care deficits. Occasionally an opportunity must be provided for acquisition of mental skills such as problem solving, or a psychomotor skill such as performing a pelvic or Pap examination. Sometimes an attitudinal change is needed, and this can often be achieved through sharing experiences in small group discussion. More often, a change in the organization of the health care system is needed to improve health and health care. A new resource could be necessary to improve health, whether new equipment, facilities, or personnel. Most often, patient behavioral change is the kind required, and skill in helping patients achieve such change is seldom the goal of many CME programs.

Planning, implementing and managing change, Step 11, is difficult; and often the change program does not achieve the levels of health and patient care desired. Sometimes the health care problem is incorrectly identified. Often the change or education program mounted is inappropriate to the problem. The health care delivery system lacks personnel skilled in planning and managing change, as well as in diagnosing the need for change. Until significantly more health professionals acquire the necessary skills to diagnose the need for change correctly and plan and manage change, this step of the Bi-Cycle Model will probably remain the most difficult to undertake.

Step 12 requires collection of data after the implementation of an appropriate change program. Also, it requires a return to the patient care cycle and a recycle beginning with Step 8.

The data of the recycling process after the change program should indicate congruency of actual practice with criterion practice. If the two practices merge, the change program has been successful; quality patient and health care has been assured. If incongruency still exists between actual practice and desired outcome, change program objectives should be reviewed and redefined, and another change program implemented.

Step 11 links the change program to the patient. The quality assurance system and the Bi-Cycle Model always begin and end with the patient. If the patient and the health team achieve the care objectives agreed to in the initial contract, the quality of health care has been assured.

If the health care objectives contracted for have not been achieved, the quality assurance system provides the opportunity to recycle through a review of the basic health care contract, the basic patient data base and health care objectives, the patient's behavior, the knowledge, skills and attitudes of the health professionals who are attempting to help the patient meet his health care goals, the health care delivery system in which all are operating, and the total resources of that system. If deficits are found in any of these system components, appropriate change programs can be planned, implemented, managed, and evaluated.

NOTES

1. C.R. Brown, Jr., and D.S. Fleisher, "The Bi-Cycle Concept—Relating Continuing Education Directly to Patient Care," *New England Journal of Medicine* 284, Supplement (May 20, 1971); also in Norman S. Stearns, ed., *Continuing Medical Education in Community Hospitals: A Manual for Program Development* (Boston: Postgraduate Medical Institute, 1971).

2. Daniel S. Fleisher *et al.* "The Mandate Project: Institutionalizing a System of Patient Care Quality Assurance," *Pediatrics* 57 (May 1976): 775-782.

Chapter 3
Medical Practice Related to Continuing Education by Practice Profiling

Sigurd E. Sivertson
and
Elaine McDonald

The quest for relevant educational objectives for the individual physician is a difficult and frustrating exercise. There are multiple reasons for this. Among them, as emphasized by Meyer,[1] is that education in medical school has not instilled into the student the ability to identify lifetime learning needs. In addition, Sivertson[2] stressed that office practice, which represents 70 to 80 percent of medical care, does not yet employ a record system that will store and retrieve information necessary for the physician to assess his or her performance and translate it into learning objectives. Furthermore, this performance is dependent on other factors (the circumstance and environment of the practice) that must be considered in planning the continuing education of a practitioner.

Although there are some systematically planned practice settings (one in Maine,[3] and another in Vermont[4]) in which these considerations and techniques are successfully employed, they are few in number. Until this type of practice setting becomes accepted and widely used, identification of individual educational needs (leading to selection of learning programs to meet those needs) will remain a difficult task.

The Department of Continuing Medical Education at the University of Wisconsin has come to this conclusion by assisting physicians in the study of their practices since 1968. The thesis has always been that practice needs and continuing education should accurately relate to each other to the benefit of the physician's patients. It is the intent here to compare and comment on the practice and continuing education profiles of 109 Wisconsin family physicians.

METHOD

The practice study method developed at the University of Wisconsin is called Individual Physician Profile (IPP) and has been described elsewhere.[5] Briefly, it provides the practicing physician with a pocket-size tape recorder on which pertinent information about each patient contact is dictated. The tape is then returned to the Department of Continuing Medical Education where the patient problems are codified into the International Classification of Diseases, Adapted (ICDA) and stored together with other information in a computer. A test generated to match this practice data is then completed by the physician. The participant is then provided a practice profile retrieved from the computer, the results of the self-assessment examination, and related recommendations for continuing education from an educational consultant.

RESULTS

Among 109 participating Wisconsin family physicians, each participant received at least one educational recommendation; some received as many as six. The average was about three. Figure 3-1 shows a comparison between the composite practice profile and the continuing medical education (CME) profile for these physicians. The top five ICDA categories, containing 61 percent of patient problems, were Category 18 (Special Conditions and Examinations Without Illness), Category 7 (Diseases of the Circulatory System), Category 8 (Diseases of the Respiratory System), Category 17 (Fractures, Trauma and Poisoning), and Category 16 (Symptoms and Ill-Defined Conditions). These same categories contained 66 percent of the recommendations for CME. Thereafter, the patient problems and recommended education were diffused throughout the remaining categories and represented a little bit of everything. No education was recommended in Category 2 (Neoplasms), which was 3 percent of the patient problems, and Category 14 (Congenital Anomalies), containing 0.5 percent of the patient problems. The configuration of the two profiles showed a degree of parallelism suggesting a significant relationship.

There were notable departures in this parallelism, however. The CME profile showed disproportionately high peaks in Categories 5 (Mental Disorders) and 7 (Diseases of the Circulatory System) and relatively less CME in Category 18 (Special Conditions and Examinations Without Illness), which held 20 percent of patient problems.

Figure 3-1

COMPARISON OF PRACTICE AND CME PROFILES
109 WISCONSIN FAMILY PRACTITIONERS

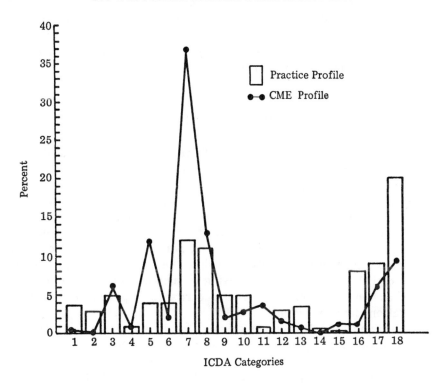

Apart from the practice profile and examination results, a more personal need was often included in the CME recommendations. This surfaced during an hour-long consultation when the educational consultant asked the question, "What types of patient problems cause you distress?" or, put another way, "If you had your choice, what patient problems would you not have come through the office door?" All participants admitted to at least one such problem and some to as many as four; the average was 1.5.

There were ten major problems causing these physicians personal distress. Psychosomatic (emotional) problems ranked number one and was cited by over half the physicians. There was a big drop to the second ranking problem, geriatrics, which was cited by almost 13 percent of the physicians. Closely following geriatrics was alcoholism and high-risk obstetrics. The remaining six patient problems (long-term illness, cardiac, diabetes, drug dependency, seriously ill children, and miscellaneous) were each cited by about 4 to 6 percent of physicians. Miscellaneous problems consisted of neurological problems, routine examinations, ill-defined conditions, auto accidents, surgical complications, chronic respiratory infections in children, patient education, glandular disturbances (endocrinology), obesity, complicated medical problems, and minor complaints.

UNDEVELOPED PHASE

It was the ultimate intent of IPP to relate continuing education to the performance of the physician and the outcome of care delivered. During the first three years, 1968-1970, the educational consultant had the opportunity to view and discuss some thirty-six participants' office records. The consultant contrasted these office records with the Problem Oriented Medical Record (POMR) of Weed,[6] which, if used correctly, makes assessment of individual performance and needs identification a part of the practice. In those years few of the physicians knew of POMR, and none was using it. The consultant's impression was that none of the existing office records would permit performance evaluation and needs identification.

Subsequently, in 1974, one motivated family physician, a member of a sophisticated group practice in a metropolitan area, agreed to use his office record to attempt such an evaluation. Together with the consultant, he reviewed the profile of his office practice in detail and selected one patient problem for which performance criteria and outcome of care would be established. The problem this physician chose was the complete annual check-up.

Standards he intended to meet for this problem were established. His secretary retrieved fourteen records of office patients who had had the complete annual check-up during the preceding months. The information recorded on the records was matched to the standards. (This was done by an independent medical record librarian from the University Hospitals.)

The result was that the record contained information matching 70 percent of his standards for performance but did not contain information pertaining to the ultimate outcome of care delivered, particularly from the patient's viewpoint. The medical record librarian, although completing the analysis, found it a most difficult and frustrating experience.

The physician accurately predicted that this would be the case, commenting, "My records are a disorganized mess." The record was indeed disorganized, and laboratory reports were stuffed in the jacket between various and sundry pages. In short, there was no systematic arrangement in his records for recording pertinent information that would permit easy use of the record for evaluation of performance. To assess thoroughness, reliability, efficiency and analytical skill was almost hopeless. The physician further stated that a major reason for this was that the physicians in the clinic could not agree on a standard format of the record, even though a patient's record was common to all of them. Each persisted in recording information according to his or her own preference. The content and organization of the patient record were not a part of their agreed-upon practice principles.

DISCUSSION

Experience with IPP has been successful—and has also fallen short of expectations. From the standpoint of success, all participants in IPP make statements similar to, "For the first time I feel that I understand my practice." In addition, all physicians perceive educational needs that relate to the problems patients bring to them. However, with a few exceptions, the process has not been able to document that either recommended education was completed or that behavior was changed as reflected in performance and outcome of care delivered.

The self-assessment examination based on the practice profile is helpful in identifying learning needs.[5] Because every physician received a different examination, test scores were not strictly comparable. Definite impressions about test results, however, can be made, and these seem to have some validity. First, those few physicians who score poorly (about 40 to 50 percent correct) do so in most of the categories, not just in one or two. Such scores strongly suggest the need for a general review and updating of knowledge. During the consultation period, the consultant is usually able to confirm this.

Second, when discussing examination results with a participant, it is usually helpful to begin with, "We've learned to use the examination results differently from how you remember test scores being used in medical school. There is no pass or fail. Let's look first at those categories where you see more patients but had 40 percent or more wrong answers. Look at Category 7...." (This was an open-ended statement to which the participant would respond.) Usually the response would take the form of, "I see a lot of patients there, and I really should have known the answer to those questions I got wrong."

In this way we attempt to bring the process of profiling and examining the participant to the point of perceiving a need directly relating to patient problems. With this as background, several of the categories representing peaks in Figure 3-1 will be discussed:

Category 7 (Diseases of the Circulatory System) ranks number one for the CME profile. There are good reasons for this:

- For one, apart from its high ranking for patient problems, a low score is even more significant because these medical problems represent a serious threat to life or quality of life.

- Second, another factor has developed concurrently with IPP and cannot be ignored in relation to diseases of the circulatory system. During this decade, technology is having a profound impact on medical care at the grass roots, e.g., intensive and coronary care units with electrocardiographic monitoring of patients. This, in turn, reflected the epidemic of ischemic heart disease and myocardial infarction in our society (about 10,000 deaths from myocardial infarction per year in Wisconsin). The need for interpreting the electrocardiogram followed in the wake of increasing sales of oscilloscopes. Physicians have to update their electrocardiographic knowledge and, in addition, teach it to nursing personnel staffing these monitoring facilities. Thus, electrocardiography is a frequent educational recommendation for these physicians and, in part, accounts for the large amount of CME in Category 7.

- Third, most of the physicians taking part in IPP have been in practice ten years or longer. Usually they score poorly on questions relating to cardiac auscultation. This is not surprising, since auscultation of the heart was not taught as effectively in the medical school curricula of past years as it is now. Thus, these physicians readily recognize a need for further knowledge and skill in that area.

- Finally, as has been pointed out in other studies of IPP, these physicians often stated: "My patients are getting older with me, I'm becoming a geriatrician." Statistics show that, in general, for every ten years these physicians had been in practice, the average age of their patients increased by five years.[7] Their geriatric profiles (patients greater than sixty-five years of age) emphasized the predominance of circulatory problems in the elderly. This, too, added to the amount of education recommended in Category 7.

As regards the disproportionately greater amount of education recommended in Category 5 (Mental Illness), this was not a direct result of the practice profile and examination results for these 109 family physicians. Instead, it is recognized during the consultation phase of IPP as the participant responds to the question about distressing patient problems. Psychosomatic or emotional types of patient problems significantly leads the list of common problems and rank far above the second most distressing problem, geriatrics. The nature of this distress usually is expressed as, "They take so much time." The reason for the excessive time in general appears to be that the practicing physician does not know how to read the unspoken language (or cues) of the patient. In part, this is a reflection of a lack of interviewing skills. The physician does not know how to ask the right questions in the right manner to get to the heart of the patient's problems expeditiously. Although there are many continuing education courses in psychiatry, there were and still are few in which the emphasis is on basic interviewing skills. Thus, a major educational need for these participants and perhaps for family practitioners in general appears to reside in this arena. Fortunately, family practice residency programs independently recognized this at the onset and emphasized interviewing skill as a strong part of their curriculum. The implication for the future is that the need for education in interviewing skills might diminish as these new residents assume their role in community medicine.

A comment about Category 2 (Neoplasms) and Category 14 (Congenital Anomalies) is in order. No education was recommended for either. This probably reflected the type of knowledge necessary to answer the test questions correctly pertaining to these two categories and is, in fact, a failure of the test bank. In general, review of the questions strongly suggested that the knowledge required was inappropriate for family practitioners and really more appropriate for physicians in tertiary care. Indirectly, therefore, it begged the question, "What knowledge and skills are required by a family practitioner in the area of neoplasms and congenital anomalies?" In-depth knowledge of pathophysiology for malignant growths and congenital anomalies seems irrelevant, if for no other reason than the fact that few patients present in a family physician's office have these types of problems. One can easily come to the conclusion that only the knowledge and skills necessary to strongly suspect malignancy or anomaly are needed. The family practitioner brings the problem to the initial level of resolution.

Category 18 (Examinations Without Illness) contains a large number of physical examinations that are done for reasons of college entrance, life insurance, well-baby and well-child, complete annual check-ups, and others. Cognitive testing in these areas represents a significant challenge. Our experience indicates that test questions probing knowledge about basic techniques of physical examination and normal anatomical variations written to simulate the environment of the physician's office serve best. Questions such as these, however, are not easily developed.

Diabetes and obesity in Category 3 ranked high as specific disease entities for all the participants in this study. In general, the participants all agreed that the need for continuing education here was minimal: the vast majority of diabetes was of the adult onset type and associated with obesity. For both this entity and obesity without diabetes, the physicians expressed resignation that there was little they could do, that they were not lacking in the required knowledge in these areas, but that the major problem was "how obese patients can be motivated to reduce their food intake." These physician participants seem to believe that the answer to that question rests in more ultimate influences that are beyond their respective domain.

Although no hard data exist, the experience of IPP tends to confirm the generally held viewpoint that the status of the patient record in office care leaves much to be desired. The example presented here is a case in point. If, as Barro[8] has stated, the patient record is the most feasible method at this time for evaluating individual physician performance, then the status of the patient record in the office becomes critical to determining education needs. Until the content and organization of information in the record are systematically arranged, thorough, reliable, and reflective of analytical skill, identification of educational needs for ambulatory care will not be feasible. Departments of continuing medical education in large centers will remain handicapped and frustrated, therefore, in their attempts to identify educational objectives. The implication is that continuing education should assist in the implementation of the patient record as a tool for making these identifications.

IPP, from the beginning, has continuously urged the development of the office record as a tool for evaluating performance in ambulatory care. More recent consultations with participants around the country indicate that the practice sector is more accepting of this and is responding to the extent that the patient office record will indeed become a dominant influence on CME in the future.

NOTES

1. T. C. Meyer, "Toward a Continuum in Medical Education," *Bulletin of the New York Academy of Medicine* 51 (June 1975): 719-726.

2. S. E. Sivertson *et al.*, "The Evaluation of Continuing Medical Education Programs," *Bulletin of the New York Academy of Medicine* 51 (June 1975): 776-784.

3. C. S. Burger, *et al.*, "Problem-Oriented Practice in Hampden Highlands, Maine," in Walker *et al.*, eds., *Applying the Problem Oriented System* (New York: Medcom Press, 1973), pp. 65-123.

4. H. M. Tufo *et al.*, "Problem Oriented Practice in Vermont," in Walker, *Ibid.*

5. S. E. Sivertson *et al.*, "Individual Physician Profile: Continuing Education Related to Medical Practice,"*Journal of Medical Education* 48 (November 1973): 1006-1012.

6. L. L. Weed, *Medical Records, Medical Education and Patient Care* (Cleveland: The Press of Case Western Reserve University, 1971).

7. S. E. Sivertson *et al.*, "The Relation Between Physician and Patient Age in Family Practice," *The Journal of Family Practice* 3 (June 1976): 305-307.

8. A. R. Barro *et al.*, "Survey and Evaluation of Approaches to Physician Performance Measurement," *Journal of Medical Education* 48 (November 1973): 1048-1090.

Chapter 4
The Physician Education Program and the Kaiser-Permanente System of Quality Assurance

Leonard Rubin

INTRODUCTION

In keeping with the theme of this volume, an attempt will be made to describe the evolution of the physician education program in the Kaiser-Permanente system of quality assurance so the policies upon which the program is now based may be more readily understood. These policies include the following:

1. Quality of care is related to education.
2. The cost of education is included as part of the cost of care.
3. Performance review (educational need assessment) is mandatory.
4. Performance review (educational need assessment) is wide based and includes such nonbiomedical aspects of medical practice as communication, time management, patient education, allied health personnel education, record keeping, self-audit, and economy of operation.
5. Mandated educational requirements are based on correcting performance deficits, not on fulfilling temporal requirements.
6. The first step in the education sequence should be problem identification rather than selection of an arbitrary topic or an arbitrary educational objective.
7. Maximum improvement in health care delivery results from the improvement in the practice of all practitioners rather than merely the elimination from practice of the tail of the Gaussian curve representing the most incompetent.
8. Modes of personal education are left to the individual physician to select. Group educational activities are selected locally.

29

THE KAISER-PERMANENTE PHYSICIAN EDUCATION PROGRAM

The following description is based primarily on activities in the Northern California Region of the Kaiser-Permanente Medical Care Program. The other five regions have similar programs that differ in a number of aspects. A programwide mandate in regard to the organizational structure of the educational program does not exist. Each region is free to establish its own mode of operation.

Within the Northern California Region, each medical center has a similar table of organization for education activity, but the educational techniques, frequency of sessions, and similar decisions are self-determined. Formal educational programs have existed in the Northern California Kaiser-Permanente Medical Care Program since its inception. Several of these programs were developed to a high level of sophistication but have been abandoned or severely reduced primarily because of apparent ineffectiveness, low cost benefit, or dwindling interest. Included in this category is a journal published many years ago, a major effort in production of audiovisual aids, and large symposia with attendance in the hundreds.

Until the latter portion of the 1960s, the programs in education consisted mainly of independent activities within each medical center with relatively little intercommunication. Inbreeding was avoided by a program in which each physician had the option of spending one-half day per week at one of the nearby academic medical centers. Because of administrative difficulties and the inequities that this option produced, it is abandoned in 1967, and a major reorganization of education was developed and implemented.

Organization

Currently the organization of the education program is as follows: All education positions are held by Permanente Group physicians who practice clinical medicine. The education program is an inherent part of operations, not an appendage. The regional coordinator of education reports directly to the executive director of The Permanente Medical Group; this is a staff position. Each of the eleven major medical centers has a physician chief of education. In addition, three of the medical centers with large house staff programs have separate directors of medical education, who have responsibility in administering the house staff program.

The major responsibilities of the regional coordinator of education include setting the budget for the regional or central operations; planning, organizing and conducting regional (interfacility) education programs; medical supervision of the regional audiovisual center; stimulation and support of innovative programs within medical centers; and management of the regional quality assurance programs. The responsibilities of the chiefs of education within each medical center include preparation of the budget within that medical center; organization of medical centerwide interdisciplinary educational programs; assisting the chief of each professional department or his designee in any of the various phases of an educational program (including establishing needs, securing educational materials, and arranging interdisciplinary activities); publishing schedules within the medical center of all educational activities; provision and maintenance of required rooms and equipment; publication of a medical center newsletter containing a variety of educational material of a biomedical, pharmaceutical, or cost containment nature; and results of quality assurance activities. In those medical centers with separate directors of medical education, the chiefs of education work closely with them to enable house staff to attend programs developed primarily for CME, and vice versa.

The regional coordinator of education conducts monthly half-day meetings attended by the chiefs of education and the directors of medical education. These meetings are concerned with educational techniques; sharing educational experiences and trials; development of regional programs; orientation of new physicians; reports from various local and national educational meetings; and education of consumers, medical students, house staff, and allied health personnel. Techniques discussed and tried have included audiovisual production, brochure and directory publication, education in management and communication techniques, as well as exchanging information concerning availability of extramural teachers and other educational techniques. Each chief of education has line responsibility to the physician-in-chief at his medical center.

Policies

The coordinator of education spends approximately 50 percent of his time on educational activities and otherwise is in practice. The chief of education in each medical center generally has a half-day per week for administration. Each has a full- or a half-time secretary. Physicians in the Medical Group have the option of one week's leave with pay for attending educational meetings. This can be accrued to two weeks. Approximately one additional hour per week of normally assigned clinic time is allowed for each physician at each medical center for educational purposes. This is usually done by the expansion of the noon-time hour on one or more occasions per week. Within each medical center there is an education committee usually chaired by the chief of education (this may or may not be different from the library committee). Each medical center has a Quality Assurance Committee separately budgeted, and in a few of the centers it is chaired by the chief of education. Additional hours (up to one half day) can be taken for this activity. Not all medical centers use this option.

There is a close liaison between the chief of education and the quality assurance chairman, if these are separate individuals; and in all cases, the chief of education is a member of the Quality Assurance Committee. Each medical center has considerable leeway in the organization of its educational activities with the exception of limits on cost and time taken from normal clinic operation. Some medical centers devote many hours to formal lectures, others relatively few. Some centers frequently invite speakers from nearby institutions, others rarely do. Educational subjects at some locations cover a wide range, from medical ethics to basic biochemistry and physiology. The range is considerably smaller in other locations and is confined to more traditional clinical subjects.

Financing

Funds for essentially all educational programs are generated from the dues paid by members of the Kaiser Foundation Health Plan. Occasionally grants from pharmaceutical or other organizations are received to augment the programs, but this represents a small portion of the total. No funding for the educational budgets comes from other Kaiser industries.

Educational budgets include the personnel costs for the coordinator of education, the chiefs of education, secretarial help, and nonpersonnel items such as supplies, audiovisual equipment, food for meetings, etc. Educational budgets do not include any compensation to nonadministrative physicians for time devoted to educational activities. There is no cost center for educational time for physicians, time for preparation for meetings, attending meetings during optional educational leave, time for making rounds in the hospital with or without house staff, or for a variety of other educational activities. These requirements are budgeted in with the overall physician requirements in the total medical care program. Medical center education budgets vary considerably from one center to another; each is determined by the chief of education and the physician-in-chief with subsequent approvals at higher levels. Allocation of funds for these budgets comes from the Kaiser Foundation Hospitals, and administration is by the physicians from The Permanente Medical Group.

Relations with Outside Organizations

All but two of the medical centers of the Kaiser-Permanente Medical Care Program in Northern California are accredited by the California Medical Association Committee on Accreditation of Continuing Medical Education. Some medical centers have approved house staff programs. In some medical centers as many as one-fifth of the physicians are involved with teaching programs in nearby academic institutions. That number is considerably lower in other locations.

Description of Programs

The spectrum of educational activities conducted on a daily basis within the Northern California Region is so wide and varied that it precludes simple classification. An attempt will be made to convey at least some appreciation for the range and number of educational programs.

Most programs at the regional level are formal and scheduled, though all do not follow traditional format. In addition to the education chiefs' monthly meeting, which deals with educational techniques as mentioned above, there are a variety of other activities. Notable is the monthly interfacility review meeting at which physicians from many specialties meet at a different medical center to audit inpatient and outpatient care with the purpose of bringing to the attention of the host institution items that they might wish to address through educational or other means to improve care. This has been in operation for four years and is quite popular.

For several years physicians in subspecialties, especially the smaller departments, have been meeting quarterly on a regional basis purely for CME purposes. These regional meetings are mostly participatory, but guest speakers are occasionally invited. These meetings are designed to avoid inbreeding of ideas in departments where opportunity does not exist for communication with sufficient numbers of peers.

Within the medical center, CME activities of a wide range occur. Lectures, seminars, courses in specific subjects, audit programs, case presentations, rounds (both inpatient and outpatient, with presentation of patients in both cases), journal clubs, clinical pathological conferences, and distribution of videotapes from the rounds held at the University of California are just a few of the formally scheduled and conducted meetings. These often involve allied health personnel. At least fifteen such programs are conducted each week at each medical center.

In addition to the formal education programs, an enormous amount of education occurs through informal educational channels. These may take the form of informal encounters and meetings between physicians in the course of seeing patients in the ambulatory area or in the hospital, seeing each others' records, seeing each others' patients while covering the hospital or clinic, and through consultations or requests for special tests. Not to be ignored is the amount of informal educational activity which is conducted because of the administrative organizational structure in which department and division heads have responsibility for the quality of care. A variety of activities and committees created for administrative purposes actually provide effective educational mechanisms.

COMMENTS AND OBSERVATIONS

In many ways the educational programs with the Kaiser-Permanente Medical Care Program are a microcosm of the educational activities on a national scale. Though certain advantages result from the high degree of organization, preplanning, and budgeting, many of the lessons learned are applicable to systems of continuing professional education of higher or lower degrees of organizational development.

Recently, considerable attention has been given nationally to the apparent lack of correlation between quality of care and education. At times this argument relates to the success of the educational process and at times to the relevance of its subject matter. Although greater or lesser degrees of subject relevance and effect on quality have been noted, not considered at all in this correlation have been many forms of education not usually included in the spectrum of educational activities. Correlation of quality of care with education usually has been limited to consideration of programmed and scheduled educational activities of the kind seen in flyers and listings. Observations made in this regard at Kaiser-Permanente clearly indicate that quality of care often improves as a result of a wide variety of nonformal CME activities such as problem identification sessions with no follow-up, individual consultation, self-review, peer pressure, normal medical administrative organizational review and control, preparation of materials for teaching, etc. The list of variable formats in which effective education is conducted is indeed lengthy. Efficacy and relevance of education in relation to quality of care should not be judged merely by those educational activities which happen to be listed on the bulletin board. It is desirable to identify, support, and assist the further development of those informal educational processes which are effective. We believe that quality care is related to education, but the whole range of educational activity must be considered to reveal the correlation.

Mandating performance review is necessary to determine deficits in quality of care. It is only in this way that most educational needs may be determined. Whether the indicated educational activity is correction of a need in knowledge, skills, or attitude must be determined by further analysis of the performance deficit found in review. Optional performance review is not consistent with good management control in any kind of business. This is no less true in the professional sphere. Optional review has been found to focus prematurely on topics or providers not necessarily in greatest need of attention. Performance review has been criticized for lack of effectiveness and lack of relevance just as other aspects of educational activity have been, and some of those criticisms are valid. However, analysis of performance review in which those criticisms are true usually reveals that a number of errors have been made. Among these is having performance review done in the "top-down" mode rather than on a "peer" mode. Even if results of such a performance review are valid, they frequently are not received properly when "handed down," and as a result desirable actions do not follow. As is true in so many areas, the marketing of performance review is extremely important. Having performance review conducted on a peer basis has multiple advantages in addition to increasing its acceptability. Performance review is in itself a valuable educational activity, not only from the point of view of discovering educational needs, but also as an effective corrective activity. To maintain the correction requires other programs that are more properly part of a quality assurance system than an educational system.

It is important to note here that performance review is not an aspect of professional life that is done normally or naturally. When it is found that it is not being performed correctly, it, too, must be taught; and the principles and practice of performance review must be included in the educational curriculum. Properly executed, performance review rapidly yields abundant evidence of deficits in quality of care with a very acceptable cost benefit.

Improvement in care following performance review frequently falters because of lack of follow-up. Systems for instituting educational activity or other corrective activity must be built into the system. If improvement is not demonstrated, the physician will classify this exercise with other so-called quality control procedures that are known to be a sham. Performance review will become a useless exercise, done in a perfunctory manner that becomes wasteful and is actually detrimental to good care because it diverts personnel and resources from direct patient management. Performance review mandated in specific topics of care in which it is actually not necessary develops into a "numbers game" in which the staff merely fills requirements and true deficits in care are not discovered. Performance review should have free range to address those areas truly in need of improvement.

Current CME is often considered to be irrelevant and ineffective in improving the quality of care because too much of it is traditionally bound to the biomedical aspects of medical practice. Most practitioners could well quote the farmer who stated in response to being offered brochures on improved farming, "I ain't farming half as good as I know how to now." Many practitioners who are found to have significant deficits in care could write acceptable treatises on the very errors in care that they have committed. Lack of biomedical knowledge is not the most frequent cause of inappropriate care. More often, it is the implementation of the knowledge which is lacking. This frequently takes the form of not knowing how to communicate (questioning, listening, or giving information), not knowing how to manage one's time, not knowing how to manage allied health personnel, or how to teach them and monitor their performance. A major problem results from poor record keeping techniques—seemingly resulting from a lack of adequate time, but actually resulting in the loss of more time. Many other areas of educational needs in the systems area apparent from performance review are not strictly within the biomedical aspects of medical practice. However, it must be realized that lack of successful educational efforts in the systems area prevents the beneficial effect of the biomedical teaching, which is so abundant. Information not used is useless. It is necessary for medical education to expand its horizons so the traditional content is given a vehicle by which it can be carried into practice. It is for these reasons that the first step in the education sequence should be problem identification rather than a priori selection of a topic.

A number of features of traditional education should be reassessed before they are permanently welded to the fabric of *continuing* medical education. High on the list of characteristics to be avoided is the fixed time program. Medical professionals above all should realize the variability among individuals. Depths of deficiencies and variable rates of learning are two factors that preclude fixed time programs. Mandating fixed time requirements for continuing medical education is perpetuating a system that should not exist even in basic medical education. Unfortunately, it has gained a foothold in CME and, because of a variety of administrative problems, is becoming the common mode. Only in recent years has there been a crack in the wall of the four-year medical school program. That wall should not be built into the area of CME. Performance review, necessary in any case for need assessment, provides an excellent tool for determining when educational requirements have been filled.

Other traditional education features to consider have to do with basic educational theory and need not be addressed in a discussion concerning public policy on CME. These have to do with curriculum formation and traditional concepts of educational objective setting.

During the course of several years of quality assessment, an interesting, useful, and originally unexpected observation has repeatedly been made during review of medical records. The number of highly significant serious errors found is relatively constant among all physicians in a setting, irrespective of their position in the hierarchy of "goodness" as determined by peer judgment. That is, "good doctors" — those most highly respected — make essentially the same number and kind of errors as those of lower stature. The reason for this is not apparent. A number of possibilities come to mind, including the greater risk and productivity of the "better" doctors, who receive rather than refer the difficult cases. At any rate, it argues against focusing review on those physicians who are believed to be poor performers.

Even if the above unexpected circumstance were not present, the mean level of medical care will be improved more by a slight improvement in all physicians than by elimination completely of the lowest few percent of physicians at the tail end of the Gaussian curve of "goodness." This latter consideration, plus the observation made above, is further argument for continued peer review for all physicians as the major thrust of the program, with focused review limited to special situations.

It is interesting to note that in performing peer review in a variety of settings such as groups, academic institutions, community hospitals, and rural and urban settings, the same relative constancy in type and numbers of indisputable deficits in care is noted, as was mentioned above in regard to physicians.

Effective quality assurance activities are associated with demonstrated and documented evidence of improvement in aspects of care that are incontrovertibly considered unacceptable by all practitioners. Sufficient numbers of gross deficits in care that will find no defenders are abundantly evident in any practice setting. The measure of success or acceptability of quality assurance and educational programs should be the numbers of these blatant errors in care which are corrected, not the number measured or attacked. Program approval by governmental and voluntary agencies should be based on improvement in performance of distinct significant aspects of care, not merely the number of medical care evaluations performed.

Because of the unique economic arrangement which exists in the Kaiser-Permanente Medical Care Program, it is difficult to extrapolate from this system to other systems in regard to funding of educational programs. This can best be discussed by others with more experience in other medical economic situations.

Chapter 5
Do Self-Assessment Methods of Continuing Medical Education Affect Quality of Patient Care?

Harold A. Zintel and
C. Rollins Hanlon

One prompt response to the question posed by the assigned title is a disappointing admission: "We don't know." It is the bias of this chapter that self-assessment methods are most likely superior to currently unpopular teaching modalities such as the lecture, but solid data to support this view are scanty. Theoretical discussions of teaching effectiveness have been or will be presented by others. This chapter will review briefly the experience of the American College of Surgeons (ACS) with its variant of the self-assessment method—the Surgical Education and Self-Assessment Program, commonly known as SESAP.

THE SESAP PROGRAM

The American College of Surgeons adopted the basic idea of its self-assessment program from that of the American College of Physicians (ACP) Medical Knowledge Self-Assessment Program. Edward C. Rosenow, Jr., as the chief executive of the ACP, provided valuable initial briefing for the regents and staff of the ACS early in 1969 and continued this helpful liaison as the original SESAP effort got underway. In addition, the consultative assistance of the National Board of Medical Examiners (NBME) has been most valuable during both the first and second SESAP efforts. For the next phase (SESAP III), however, the American College of Surgeons plans to develop its own in-house educational consultants, both full- and part-time, recognizing that they will be building on the experience gained from the association with the NBME, along with the ACP.

SESAP I was introduced in the fall of 1971. It was based on the same premises as the Medical Knowledge Self-Assessment Program of the

ACP: aiming at the needs of the learners, rather than the desires or opinions of the continuing education committee. A desire for continuing learning by physicians was assumed, at least by those physicians who would enroll in the program. It was also assumed that physicians were willing to identify their deficiencies in knowledge and technique as long as no one else, especially the government, was aware of these defects. ACS remains convinced that they are willing to assess themselves voluntarily if it can be done at their own convenience with assurance that the individual results will remain confidential.

The confidentiality of the enterprise was dictated, not only by the natural desire of every individual to keep his deficiencies secret, but specifically by a widespread concern during the late 1960s and early 1970s that unsatisfactory performance might be cited by federal agencies or others as a basis for control or restriction of surgical practice. Therefore, ACS went to great lengths to assure its fellowship that their individual performance would be known only to them, and that no record would be kept of their participation. With the current insistence on credit for educational experiences, the latter condition might now appear bizarre. But concern over invasion of privacy was intense at the time, and absolute confidentiality was considered essential, regardless of consequences such as loss of useful data for educational research. In later editions of SESAP, ACS has not used the bonded mailing agency to separate the recordkeeping entirely from college files. The confidentiality of individual performance is preserved, but there is a record of participation.

SESAP I was constructed by the Committee on Continuing Education, along with NBME and forty-four additional surgeons representing general surgery and the ten other surgical specialties. Essentially, it was a self-administered, voluntary assessment process; scrupulous efforts to avoid labeling it an "examination" were made to circumvent the connotation of passing or failing grades. Moreover, the scorable units of the process were not "questions" but "items." These conventions in terminology were considered important in emphasizing the educational character of the effort, rather than having it considered as a test. Assessment was available if the participant wished to have it but was not compulsory for those enlisting in the exercise. As others have pointed out elsewhere, one is more likely to gain full benefit from such an experience by setting a goal of behavior modification tied to the feedback mechanism of assessment against norms.

Seven hundred fifty clinically oriented "objective" items comprised SESAP I, covering the broad field of surgery and emphasizing new information which might have developed since the practicing surgeon completed his residency some five or ten years earlier. An attempt was made to cover that body of knowledge considered essential for all surgeons, whether in the specialty of general surgery or in other specialties. Seven categories of the program were:

1. Cardiovascular and respiratory;
2. Musculoskeletal and neurosurgical;
3. Skin, breast and burns;
4. Gastrointestinal surgery;
5. Genitourinary and gynecologic surgery;
6. Metabolism, shock and endocrine surgery; and
7. Head, neck, ear, nose, throat and ophthalmology.

In addition, items related to cancer and to trauma were dispersed throughout the other categories and were capable of separate consideration in overall analysis.

One of the critical areas in design of the program is the level of sophistication or depth probed by the items. The committee attempted to address a certain body of knowledge that surgeons of all types should possess if they are to administer competent surgical care. Detailed assessment of highly technical knowledge required in various specialty fields was to be left to the specialties themselves. This might be addressed by their "in-training examinations," administered repetitively at various levels in the graduate training programs of each specialty, or by the examination of the specialty boards for certification.

In addition to SESAP and the examinations sponsored by individual specialties, one should mention the "Basic Surgical Examination" generated under the auspices of the American Board of Medical Specialties as a common denominator or "core content" of all surgery. It had been conceived as a possible common Part One for the generally two-stage examination of each surgical specialty. This rational, effort-saving mechanism was constructed by all the surgical specialties, including general surgery, working in concert. But lack of uniform support by the parent bodies has gradually brought it to the edge of dissolution. Its history is an unfortunate monument to inadequate cooperation.

Returning to SESAP, its scoring mechanism was the decile rating system, anticipating that the surgical knowledge of the participants would vary according to a normal frequency distribution curve. It was assumed that those who scored in the lowest deciles, compared with peers in their own specialty, might personally interpret this as a need for additional effort in a given area of knowledge. The original plan, difficult to implement for specific individuals except through their own choice, was for the college to offer at its spring meeting an appropriate series of intensive seminars stressing individual participation in courses oriented toward problem-solving under supervision. These courses would be programmed after review of computer patterns pointing out areas of widespread, inadequate performance.

It is not necessary to detail every aspect of the SESAP mechanism, which has been well spelled out in publications sponsored by the college[1] or by the president of the NBME.[2] After each category of items, there are bibliographic references, keyed to individual items. The individual can take the program by the closed-book or the open-book method; if the former, during a specified early phase of the program, his performance is included in the computer determined norms, against which he can score his performance by referring to the answer key provided. If one looks up the reference before he answers, the scoring obviously has no meaning but the amplification of knowledge is presumably accomplished.

Enrollment in SESAP I continued for three years and enlisted some 15,000 participants. SESAP II was introduced in mid-1974 after three years of preparation at the hands of seventy authorities in surgical and medical science and in educational methodology. The cutoff date for computer scoring was early 1975, following which self-scoring was again employed. After the development of the computer norms for SESAP II, a syllabus of critiques was made available to all enrollees, including those who had already completed the assessment items. This was essentially a 500-page textbook of surgery, containing not only the 750 items but also a discussion critique of each item with the so-called correct answer and appropriate references for further reading. There is, in addition, a service by the John Crerar Library in Chicago for obtaining reprints of the cited references. This service is currently in question as to its applicability because of recent changes in copyright legislation.

To date, over 29,000 SESAP I and II packets have been distributed. SESAP II will continue to be offered until the initiation of SESAP III in October 1979. This offering will precede the first voluntary recertification process of the American Board of Surgery in 1980. Presumably, the recertification will be based not only on an examination of knowledge but also on performance criteria such as evidence of continuing educational effort, and possibly practice audit. Potential candidates for recertification will be advised that SESAP II and SESAP III, plus other material provided in educational offerings by the American College of Surgeons, form a base of information useful in preparation for the recertification process.

EVALUATION

It is apparent that SESAP measures knowledge and not clinical competence. The latter is presumably the vital factor affecting quality of patient care, contingent on a combination of knowledge, clinical experience, technical skill, and the imponderable component of judgment. Performance by junior surgical trainees, short on experience but long on information and familiarity with challenging examinations, might surpass that of ostensibly competent senior clinicians. This is an issue highly relevant to the question posed by the title of this chapter. SESAP II has made the assumption, in the words of a previous chairman of ACS's Continuing Education Committee, James V. Maloney, Jr., that "given two surgeons of equal intellectual capacity, experience, and technical skill, the more knowledgeable surgeon will provide better patient care. Until a better measure of clinical competence is developed, this assumption alone justifies the effort on the part of the surgeon to evaluate and expand his own knowledge."

Whether self-assessment methods of continuing medical education affect quality of patient care is part of the larger question of the role of any formal education in affecting patient care. Maloney's assumption has been cited; without expanding on it unduly, one should mention simply that it is difficult to recognize and treat satisfactorily a clinical entity with which one is totally unfamiliar.

It would be easy to cite the conclusions of the preceding and following chapters, reviewing the Bi-Cycle concept, the importance of motivation toward lifetime learning instilled at the medical school level or earlier, and the recognition that physicians must somehow infuse each day's clinical experience with a learning component. No claim is made that SESAP simulates exactly the audit-stimulated and guided correction of variations from acceptable clinical performance, as occurs with personal supervision of a colleague's performance. However, it appears to approach such simulation of clinical experience, especially if it incorporates the newer techniques based on branching logic.

Whether it would be possible to design an educational experiment to test the effect of such self-assessment on the quality of patient care is problematical. However, if one added such an experimental design to the basic costs of SESAP on its current scale, it does not seem that the examination would remain within the affordable range.

NOTES

1. W.S. Blakemore and J.V. Maloney, Jr., "The Surgical Education and Self-Assessment Program," *Bulletin of the American College of Surgeons* 56 (June 1971): 9.

2. John P. Hubbard, "Self-Education and Self-Assessment as a New Method for Continuing Medical Education," *Archives of Surgery* 103 (September 1971): 422-424.

Part II
Required Systems of CME Programs

Chapter 6
Reexamination/Recertification: Measurement of Professional Competence and Relation to Quality of Medical Care

Robert A. Chase and
Fredric D. Burg

In the title used in this discussion, the word "reexamination" is used. All too commonly the word examination is defined in a limited way. To many, examination means a paper and pencil exam. Therefore, we would much prefer to use the term "evaluation," since evaluation, both voluntary and mandatory, may take many forms, including:

1. Traditional examinations
   Paper and pencil — multiple choice question or essay
   Patient-management problems
   Oral examinations

2. Computer-based examination

3. Simulation models and audiovisual simulation

4. Audit
   Audit of behavior — behavioral checklists
   Audit of record
   Self-audit by questionnaire
   Assessment of outcome

5. Peer Review — foundations or Professional Standards Review Organizations

6. Appraisal by seniors

7. Educational background

8. Resume of past performance

EVALUATION METHODOLOGY

It is not within the scope of this chapter to address the many complex issues related to evaluation methodology. However, a few general comments could be helpful as background for the discussion that follows. First, the various methods outlined above reflect multiple strategies or approaches to evaluation. Perhaps this concept can best be described by considering the several dichotomies represented among the methods cited:

- Process vs. outcome
- Direct vs. indirect
- Prospective vs. retrospective
- Fixed point vs. continuing
- Real vs. simulated

Obviously, the decision to use a particular method must be made in relation to the objective it is intended to serve. Such decisions must also recognize that each approach and each method have inherent strengths and limitations. Then, there is the practical consideration that certain methods, such as the traditional multiple-choice examination, are already available, whereas others, such as the computer-based examination, are still in development. Finally, it is important to remember that each evaluation methodology outlined above measures only some elements of total "physician competence." It is equally important to remember that physician competence is but one important element of total "health care quality."

That much-used, much-abused generic term, "health care quality," is inserted into so many arenas today that it is beginning to lose its impact, if not its credibility. Donabedian's complex frame of reference or construct for health care quality displays the complexity of its definition.[1] Health care quality *is* difficult to define and beyond our ability to measure as an entity. Nevertheless, we hear the argument that there is no *evidence* or *proof* that continuing medical education affects "health care quality." There is also apparently no proof that violence on our television affects the crime rate. In both instances, lack of proof is itself no proof that there is no effect. Since, as far as we are aware, there is no proof that continuing medical education has *no* effect on health care quality, We suggest that it is reasonable to assume that it does and will continue to have a positive effect.

We endorse Mildred Moorehead's comment:"There is a great deal that can be done in this country today to upgrade current practice without the need to defer until science has definite proof for all the modalities in use."[2] All the odds are in favor of a positive effect on health care quality by the participation of physicians in CME.

There are at least three other major variables — patient and family attitudes, demographic variables, and quality in health care facilities — that would have a major influence on the quality of care provided to an individual. Focusing in on the role of the physician in this particular model, one notes that physician performance is most likely dependent on physician knowledge, skills, and abilities, which are again most likely dependent on a variety of educational and learning experiences. Thus, to draw conclusions about physician competency on the basis of the quality of care provided to a patient is a complicated task. It is possible that because of the potential strength of these nonphysician variables, they could result in an inaccurate judgment concerning physician competency, if quality of care is used as a sole criterion.

The National Board of Medical Examiners is involved in strategies to develop methods of measuring the important components of competency of physicians, components that contribute to high quality health care. Every responsible evaluation agency is very much involved in determining the validity of available evaluation methods. Does the instrument measure a competency that is relevant to the physician's ability to perform his role in an effective way? Do physicians who perform well on the evaluation actually perform better in practice than those who perform poorly on the evaluation? Is there a point or standard in performance on the evaluation that is so low that the physician is considered *not* competent to practice?

If the answer to this last question is in the affirmative, one simply (actually *not* so simply) must decide what that low point is. Once the standard is set, agencies acting in the public interest will have a "cause for action" a physician will be licensed or denied a license. One must use "cause for action" with care because there is no absolute proof that a person scoring at a certain level will always perform with competence in a general sense. He or she merely demonstrates a capability for competence in those areas measured by the evaluation instrument. To the extent that competence in those measurable areas is essential to the safe, independent practice of medicine, demonstrated lack of this capability should deny a physician the right to unrestricted practice. This is not to ignore the fact that many competencies important to the safe practice of medicine are *not* measurable. For example, honesty, motivation, humanism and interpersonal skills are not yet subject to reliable objective assessment. This does not relieve society of the responsibility for using some form of evaluation of these qualities—such as evaluations from teachers, supervisors or peers—recognizing, however, the limitations of such subjective judgments.

Nonetheless, one is haunted by the competencies that are not subject to objective measurement, and the result is a constant prod to the profession to continue the research activities that are generating new methodology for evaluation of these other elements of competence.

At the same time, our present limitation in the noncognitive domain does not relieve the profession of the responsibility for measuring those competencies that are reliably measurable. The importance of the cognitive base cannot be outweighed by interpersonal skills and motivation. The knowledgeable physician deficient in "caring" is admittedly incompetent, but the "caring" physician without knowledge is dangerous.

Other chapters address the various incentive-disincentive mechanisms other than reexamination (reevaluation) and recertification that motivate physicians to participate in CME. This chapter will center on the areas of reexamination and recertification.

At the outset one should stress that reexamination *alone* is unlikely to serve as the sole basis for recertification—any more than examination *alone* has provided the sole basis for licensure or specialty certification. State boards license physicians and specialty boards certify specialists only after educational requirements are satisfied, recommendation is made, and the candidate is evaluated by examination.

Rosemary Steven's book, *American Medicine and the Public Interest*,[3] and more recently Robert Richard's thesis, "Current Forces Influencing Continuing Medical Education in the United States,"[4] trace the development of specialty boards and licensure. Together with many supporting publications, they display the positive effects on health care quality by elimination of unqualified charlatans through licensure. Similarly, it can be expected that *re*licensure and *re*certification will help to protect the public against possible erosion of competence over time of licensed and certified physicians.

First, some facts on the history of development of specialty certification:

1. In the pre-Flexnerian era, graduate medical education varied in quality, was largely entrepreneurial, and was chaotic.
2. Although apprenticeship experiences existed in the nineteenth century (in fact, the Pennsylvania Hospital has employed graduate trainees since its founding in 1751), residency-style training in the modern sense started at Johns Hopkins Hospital in 1889.

3. By 1914, 70 percent of medical school graduates were taking internships. There were 3,000 internships for 3,500 U.S. medical graduates at that time.

4. Specialty societies, like the American College of Surgeons and the American College of Physicians, emerged; in 1916, the American Board of Ophthalmology, the first specialty board, was established.

5. In 1919, eighteen graduate schools of medicine were recognized by the Council of Medical Education.

6. The rest of the story has been incremental emergence of specialty boards in each practice discipline, until at present there are twenty-two such certifying agencies.

7. In 1930, the Advisory Board of Medical Specialties was established as a common organization for specialty boards and associated organizations. It was reorganized in 1970 to become the American Board of Medical Specialties.

The effect on the educational programs has been predictably positive, and the health care of individuals almost certainly has been improved as highly trained specialists have emerged from the certification system. More controversial is the current trend of certification of individuals in narrow *sub*disciplines, such as neonatal and perinatal medicine, gynecologic oncology, dermatopathology, medical nuclear physics, etc. There are currently general or special certificates in sixty-five areas of medical practice. Certification might be justified in these areas, but at some point such certification becomes counterproductive in terms of meeting health care needs of the public at large.[5] There are at least eighteen additional special competency areas that can be expected to apply to the American Board of Medical Specialties for special competence certification. Recognizing that the system has produced highly trained and skilled specialists, there is nonetheless concern that the system could be unresponsive to societal needs.

Specialty training is now an integral part of medical education for essentially all physicians. The Tracking Study by Levit and Associates that followed the graduating medical class of 1960 pointed out that by 1972, 99 percent of the graduates had completed at least two years of postgraduate training, 86 percent had completed residency programs, and 73 percent were by then board certified.[6] With the establishment of the American Board of Family Practice in 1969, all fields of medical practice are now recognized within the specialty board structure, and it is logical to predict that most U.S. medical graduates will be certified in the years ahead.

Leading to this phenomenon has been the tremendous growth in the number of residency training programs from 1930 to the present. In 1930, there were 2,028 residency positions in 338 hospitals. By 1955, that number had reached 25,841 in 1,201 hospitals. At present, there are 65,357 in 4,840 hospital-based approved programs. Of the 65,357 positions offered in 1975, 91 percent were filled positions. Thirty-one percent were filled by foreign medical graduates. The National Intern Resident Matching Program data for 1976 show that a total of 16,112 first-year positions were offered and that 76 percent were filled by the matching system. Of interest is the·fact that of the 9,060 positions offered in the primary care specialties (family practice, internal medicine, pediatrics and obstetrics and gynecology), 87 percent were filled; but in the nonprimary care specialties only 55 percent were filled through the Intern Resident Matching Plan.

The principle of *re*certification makes the same sense that *re*licensure does in terms of the public's protection against incompetence. The idea that a physician's competence might not decay if it remains unattended is senseless. One-time licensure *or* one-time specialty certification is equally senseless as long as licensure or certification by law or by precedent is a permit to take the responsibility for care of an ill patient.

The specialty boards generally recognize the logic of recertification. A committee of the American Board of Medical Specialties (ABMS) recommended recertification in 1940, but it was not until 1973 that the ABMS adopted recertification as a principle for all boards. All twenty-two specialty boards now endorse the concept of recertification. Several of the boards have instituted or are about to institute voluntary recertification strategies. The newest specialty board, the American Board of Family Practice (ABFP), declared from its inception that recertification shall be mandatory. The ABFP limited the period of certification to six years, with examination essential for continued certification. The first mandatory recertification program for ABFP will start in 1977. Meanwhile, other specialty boards have instituted voluntary recertification, starting with the American Board of Internal Medicine, which held its first voluntary recertification examination in October 1974. About 3300 diplomates took the one-day examination.

The following specialty boards have set target dates for recertification as follows:

American Board of Internal Medicine   1974
American Board of Family Practice   1976

American Board of Physical Medicine and Rehabilitation	1977
American Board of Ob-Gyn	1977-78
American Board of Allergy and Immunology	1978
American Board of Nuclear Medicine	1978
American Board of Plastic Surgery	1978
American Board of Radiology	1978
American Board of Otolaryngology	1978
American Board of Surgery	1985
American Board of Colon and Rectal Surgery	1985
American Board of Thoracic Surgery	1986
American Board of Ophthalmology	date not set

The major generic influences on development of recertification and participation in CME are public accountability and the public and profession's recognition of the perishability of medical knowledge.

Recertification is now at the stage of development where certification found itself in 1920, and CME finds itself where graduate education was at about the same time. This prospect of recertification has had enormous impact on the behavior of the professions, as evidenced by the success of self-assessment examinations, the attendance at CME meetings, and the increased use of other CME tools by the professions. The AMA has accredited CME programs for fifteen years; during that time the number of courses has more than tripled, and registrations have quintupled. How much such participation in continuing medical education and self-assessment will change physician behavior and thereby the quality of practice remains difficult to measure. But one can assume that there is a positive change in overall physician competence by the upgrading of some components of competence through CME. One cannot *prove* an effect on the "quality of care," but every element of common sense suggests that the modular improvement that occurs colors the whole quality of care — unmeasurable as it may be.

It is timely to examine the influences both driving and restraining the development of recertification by specialty boards. Richards, in his thesis on CME, uses the force-field strategy to display influences on CME.[2] I shall use the same method to serve as a focus for discussion of incentive and disincentive forces on recertification. Figure 6-1 displays such individual influences.

The strength of the various forces involved is to some extent dependent upon the size of the stick or the attractiveness of the carrot carried by the responsible agency. Policy makers must consider incentive carrots to the profession in addition to the obvious sticks. The mechanisms by which agencies influence recertification are shown in Table 6-1.

Figure 6-1

FIELD FORCE DIAGRAM: INCENTIVES AND DISINCENTIVES ON RECERTIFICATION

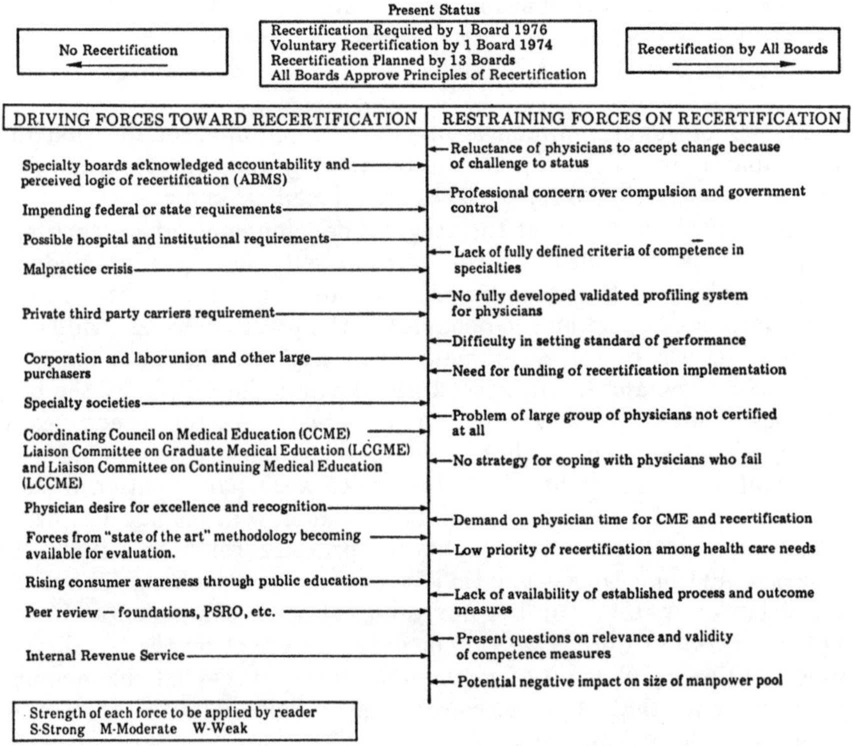

	Present Status Recertification Required by 1 Board 1976 Voluntary Recertification by 1 Board 1974 Recertification Planned by 13 Boards All Boards Approve Principles of Recertification	
No Recertification		Recertification by All Boards

DRIVING FORCES TOWARD RECERTIFICATION	RESTRAINING FORCES ON RECERTIFICATION
Specialty boards acknowledged accountability and perceived logic of recertification (ABMS)	←Reluctance of physicians to accept change because of challenge to status
Impending federal or state requirements	←Professional concern over compulsion and government control
Possible hospital and institutional requirements	
Malpractice crisis	← Lack of fully defined criteria of competence in specialties
Private third party carriers requirement	←No fully developed validated profiling system for physicians
	←Difficulty in setting standard of performance
Corporation and labor union and other large purchasers	←Need for funding of recertification implementation
Specialty societies	
Coordinating Council on Medical Education (CCME) Liaison Committee on Graduate Medical Education (LCGME) and Liaison Committee on Continuing Medical Education (LCCME)	←Problem of large group of physicians not certified at all
	←No strategy for coping with physicians who fail
Physician desire for excellence and recognition	←Demand on physician time for CME and recertification
Forces from "state of the art" methodology becoming available for evaluation.	←Low priority of recertification among health care needs
Rising consumer awareness through public education	
Peer review — foundations, PSRO, etc.	←Lack of availability of established process and outcome measures
Internal Revenue Service	← Present questions on relevance and validity of competence measures
	← Potential negative impact on size of manpower pool

Strength of each force to be applied by reader S-Strong   M-Moderate   W-Weak

Table 6-1

INFLUENCES ON RECERTIFICATION

Agency or Factor	Mechanisms
Specialty board and ABMS	1. Board membership in ABMS dependent upon its recertification requirement 2. Directory of medical specialists; listing of recertification dates. 3. Limited period of certification

Table 6-1 (Continued)

Agency or Factor	Mechanisms
Federal government	1. Physician service reimbursement—government programs 2. Hospital restriction via hospital reimbursement—Joint Commission on Accreditation of Hospitals (JCAH) and hospital privileges 3. National licensure
State government	1. Physician service reimbursement 2. Licensure and relicensure via certification and recertification 3. Appointment to health care panels
Hospital or institution, i.e., school of medicine	1. Hospital privileges 2. Institutional appointments 3. Physician service reimbursement 4. Make preparation (CME) available and accessible
Malpractice crisis	1. Insurability 2. Premium costs 3. Deterrant or incentive of liability threat
Private third party carriers	1. Physician service reimbursement 2. Advertise participating physicians
Corporations, labor unions and other large purchasers	1. Physician service reimbursement 2. Appointment to panels
Specialty societies	1. Condition of continuing membership 2. Make self-assessment and CME available
CCME—LCGME & LCCME	1. Approval of program only where faculty is recertified 2. Urge increase priority of recertification
The certified physician	1. Motivation of profession and acceptance by profession 2. Awareness of own deficiencies by self-assessment and self-audit 3. Awareness of own deficiencies by performance profile—Quality Assurance Program, PSRO, etc.
Testing agencies in cooperation with specialty boards	1. Assure validity of evaluation strategies 2. Develop fully profiling system for physicians 3. Evolve competency displays for specialties 4. Produce new methodology for evaluation of process—outcome

Table 6-1 (Continued)

Agency or Factor	Mechanisms
	5. Develop rational standard setting mechanisms
Organized medicine	1. Persuade profession to accept logic of recertification
	2. Design mechanism for coping with physicians who are substandard
	3. Aid in funding CME and recertification costs
	4. Faster reorganization of health care delivery to free physician time
	5. Augment priority of CME and recertification
	6. Evolve system to motivate noncertified to be certified or at least to participate in recertification program
Joint Commission on Accreditation of Hospitals (JCAH)	1. Accreditation of institutions only with defined hospital privileges
	2. Accreditation of institutions only with programs of CME
Peer review—PSRO	1. Require physician to perform at level to meet criteria
Internal Revenue Service	1. CME costs deductible for physician

All of the agencies mentioned in Table 6-1 ought to participate in financing of preparation for recertification through CME strategies and Self-Assessment Systems as well as in the initial start-up cost of recertification, when necessary.

FORCES INFLUENCING RECERTIFICATION

Specialty boards working as a consortium through the ABMS first considered a recommendation for recertification in 1940. Currently, the concept of recertification is endorsed by all specialty boards, and the ABMS has promulgated guidelines on recertification:

1. Recertification should assure, through periodic evaluations, the physician's continuing competence in his chosen area of specialty practice.

2. Recertification should encourage certified physicians to continue those educational activities essential to the maintenance of competence in their specialties.

3. It is the prerogative of individual boards to elect voluntary or mandatory recertification; however, a specialty board may not rescind initial certificates by recertification procedures unless a date of expiration was a condition of the original certification.

4. Similar intervals for recertification by the specialty boards are desirable; an appropriate interval appears to be six years but not more than ten.

5. Upon recertification, the listing of a specialist in the *Directory of Medical Specialists* will include the date of original certification and the dates of any recertifications.

6. Recertification can apply to any of the fields in which a specialty board grants certificates.

7. Member boards are encouraged to develop procedures for recertification that are most appropriate to the characteristics of their specialty practice. Evaluated participation in continuing education, oral or written cognitive examinations, skills and performance evaluations, practice audits, and practice profiles are among the elements that should be considered and utilized as may be appropriate and with suitable emphasis or weighting.

8. Policies and procedures for recertification should be incorporated in the published requirements for certification provided by each specialty board.

9. In the light of rapid developments now taking place in examination and testing technics, member boards are also encouraged to review on a continuing basis the recertification procedures they might develop and adopt.

10. The design of recertification procedures requires close collaboration between specialty boards and their related specialty societies and other constituencies; however, the determination of policies and procedures affecting the recertification process is ultimately the responsibility of each primary or conjoint board.

One mechanism the ABMS may use to influence boards to develop systems of recertification is continuing membership in ABMS by a member board. The boards themselves may follow the lead of the American Board of Family Practice and limit the period of active certification, thereby making recertification mandatory. The ABMS will include dates of certification and recertification in the *Directory of Medical Specialists*. This will likely influence individuals to recertify.

Federal and State Governments

The federal government is likely to restrict reimbursement for services to patients under federal programs to individual providers with proper certification. This is particularly true when the service is complex and logically requires the service of a specialist. Several bills under study in committee during the last few years have included provisions incorporating this principle. It is natural to assume that, like certification, recertification might be required for reimbursement once such a policy is established.

Operating through pressure on the JCAH or directly, the federal government could insist that physicians' privileges in hospitals depend on physician certification and, ultimately, recertification. The mechanism for control would be reimbursement to hospitals for patient services to patients under federal programs such as Medicare and Medicaid. Some bills proposed by influential federal legislators include recommendations for federal licensure with federally established standards. It is a predictable next step that certification and recertification might be federalized.

Some state governments are likely to broaden their existing policies to reimburse for state-funded special services only to certified physicians. State crippled children services, for example, commonly insist on care by certified specialists if services are to be covered. The logical next step is that recertification is likely to be insisted on as well, whether or not the specialty board itself makes it mandatory.

A growing number of states have relicensure requirements at present. This could be stimulated further if the current federal Senate Health manpower bill passes. Senator Edward Kennedy's subcommittee on health recommends that states be given grants if they wish to implement "model" relicensure programs. It is a natural conclusion that some states will accept recertification as one means of acquiring automatic relicensure.

Institutional Requirements

Hospitals on their own, or as a requirement for accreditation by JCAH or for certification by the state, already limit certain hospital privileges to certified physicians. Hospital-based physicians and physicians contracted with for hospital services commonly must be certified. In each case, continuing relationship to the hospital could require recertification on a regular basis. Hospitals create an incentive for physicians to participate in CME and recertification by making continuing education programs readily available and by requiring physician participation for continuing staff membership.

Malpractice

The malpractice situation is a strong incentive to physicians to hold unassailable credentials. The 1973 report by the HEW commission on medical malpractice had as its top recommendation periodic relicensing of physicians based on proof of participation in approved CME programs, as well as a recommendation for periodic reevaluation and recertification of physicians by their specialty boards. With the liability principle of "hospital responsible for care of its patients," hospitals have a strong incentive to insist on up-to-date credentials as a requirement for staff membership and privileges.

The 1975 Michigan law relating to malpractice has tough provisions on relicensure. Certification and recertification cannot be far behind as possible requirements under state malpractice statutes.

Since the importance of the "locality rule" is diminishing as it applied to malpractice litigations, national standards of care by specialty will apply in all areas. This will further prompt hospitals to insist on certification and recertification for staff privileges and will prompt individual physicians to have these credentials in order. C. B. Chapman, at the Anglo-American Congress on CME stated: "Some physicians have lost malpractice suits specifically because it was shown in court that they had made no effort to keep up by reading or by some form of continuing education on a regular basis."[8] What better proof of this will there be than failure to recertify. Chapman continues, "A constant record of regular and frequent attendance at continuing or postgraduate educational courses, and willingness to seek recertification, are the best conceivable evidence of intent."

Malpractice insurance carriers are also likely to insist on recertification for continuing liability coverage for physicians.

Professional Group Standards

The Coordinating Council on Medical Education (CCME), working through its Liaison Committee on Graduate Medical Education (LCGME), could also exert pressure on residency programs to encourage or even require recertification of teaching staff. Through its Liaison Committee on Continuing Medical Education (LCCME), the CCME will influence CME programs and generate an incentive for the profession to participate in CME and self-assessment, which ultimately moves physicians toward recertification.

Third Party Carriers

Private third party carriers have the powerful incentive — reimbursement for professional services — with which to insist on credentials of providers. Most health plans reimburse at a higher level for services rendered by certified specialists over noncertified physicians. Obviously the same may apply to *re*certification. Carriers could also insist that participating physicians be certified. Since carriers release names of "participating" physicians to the public (indirect advertising), a possibly strong incentive for certification and recertification exists.

Just as third party insurance carriers influence physicians to acquire credentials through reimbursement and membership, so also could large corporations and unions and other large purchasers of medical care.

Specialty Societies

Specialty societies sometimes make certification a condition of membership, and there is every reason to believe that continuing membership would require *re*certification. The specialty societies have a major incentive role in recertification by making self-assessment and continuing education readily available, attractive, and even a condition for continuing membership.

Individual Physicians

Physicians themselves commonly possess a strong desire for excellence, gain intrinsic enjoyment from acquiring new and useful knowledge, and sometimes crave recognition. The success of the American Medical Association's Physician Recognition Award is in part a response to those intrinsic physician drives. There are now more than 40,750 physicians who hold a Physician's Recognition Award.

A certified physician can become aware of his deficiencies by participation in a self-assessment examination or by a performance profile developed through various quality assurance programs such as PSRO. Once a physician is aware, he or she should have a strong drive to learn and then be recognized by recertification.

Organized Medicine

One deterrent to physician acceptance of CME, relicensure, and recertification is the question of the validity of the evaluation strategies and the application of these strategies for purposes of making pass/fail decisions about the physician in practice for many years. It is a serious obligation of testing agencies, in cooperation with specialty boards, to assure validity of evaluation measures by acceptable educational psychology methods (evaluate the evaluation), and more fully to develop profiling systems for practicing physicians. Profiling in this context means the ability of an evaluation system to be capable of assessing a physician's competency in relationship to his own day-to-day activities in practice. Evaluation methods should be competency-based and should measure competence by evaluation not only of knowledge and problem-solving capability but also of the process of care by the physician and by the outcome. Specialty boards and professional evaluation experts together must assure that standard-setting for recertification is rational and fair.

Organized medicine has a capital role in influencing recertification. To carry out its prime role of persuading the profession at large that recertification is logical and sensible, organized medicine must display to the profession its own assignment of high priority to CME and recertification. It must design mechanisms for coping with physicians who are substandard. An organization can augment the reorganization of medical practice in ways that will free physicians for participation in programs leading to recertification. Medical organizations already spend large amounts of money on CME. They may even help finance the cost of recertification. Finally, such groups can evolve systems to motivate noncertified physicians to become certified or, as a minimum, to participate in programs that prepare physicians for recertification.

ENABLING RECERTIFICATION

Over the past half decade, there has been an increment in forces moving the profession toward recertification and a decrement in the restraining forces. The whole process will be catalyzed by available funding through grants to implement start-up CME, development of performance- and competency-based assessment measures, and recertification. Specialty boards serving relatively small numbers of candidates have serious difficulty funding certification—to say nothing of recertification. An adequate mechanism to implement recertification can emerge only from the profession itself, working through the ABMS and specialty boards. The means to discharge this responsibility reasonably should at the outset come from public and private sources. Eventually the system can become self-supporting through evaluation and certification fees.

The public interest will be served best when there are adequate mechanisms to assess continuing competence of all physicians. As a minimum, there must be a system to guard against incompetence through obsolescence of any of the practicing professionals.

NOTES

1. Avedis Donabedian, "A Perspective of Concepts of Health Care Quality," Institute of Medicine Occasional Paper, November 6-7, 1974.

2. Mildred Moorehead, "Comment and Dissent Advancing the Quality of Health Care," Institute of Medicine Publication Number 74-04 (Washington: National Academy of Sciences, 1974).

3. Rosemary Stevens, *American Medicine and the Public Interest* (New Haven, Conn., and London, England: Yale University Press, 1971).

4. Robert Richards, "Current Forces Influencing Continuing Medical Education in the United States," Ph.D. Thesis, University of Michigan (Ann Arbor, Michigan: University Microfilms, 1975).

5. Robert A. Chase, "Proliferation of Certification in Medical Specialties: Productive or Counterproductive?", *New England Journal of Medicine* 294, no. 9 (1976): 497-499.

6. E. J. Levit, M. Sabshin, and C. B. Mueller, "Trends in Graduate Medical Education and Specialty Certification: A Tracking Study of U.S. Medical School Graduates," *New England Journal of Medicine* 290 (March 1974): 545-549.

7. Richards, *op. cit.*

8. Carleton B. Chapman, "The Future of Continuing Education in the United States: A Pragmatic View," in *Proceedings of Anglo American Conference on Continuing Medical Education* (London: The Royal Society of Medicine, 1974), pp. 106-109.

Chapter 7
Recertification in Family Practice

J. Jerome Wildgen

The designation "certified specialist" applies to this author for only six years. In 1976 the American Board of Family Practice will give its first recertification exam to diplomates originally certified in 1970. Because diplomate status is certified by the American Board of Family Practice (ABFP) for only a six-year period (with a one-year grace period to complete recertification), there will be a recertifying exam each year for diplomates who were originally certified for six, or in some cases seven, years previously.

CME AND RECERTIFICATION: THE CONCEPT

The concept of mandatory CME hours as a requirement for membership in a specialty society originated with the birth of the American Academy of General Practice (AAGP) in 1948. An arbitrary decision was made to require 150 hours of CME every three years for recertification for membership in the American Academy. This requirement has remained constant throughout the years, though there has been a reclassification of the nature of the 150 hours every three years to tighten control of the content. At the present time, the documented 150 hours must include seventy-five hours of prescribed credit, which are closely controlled and approved programs or courses by the Commission on Education of the American Academy. This control was originated to improve the quality and relevance of the CME programs presented to family physicians by the various providers. Mandatory CME was an innovation in the medical profession in 1948, and this has evolved into similar requirements by numerous other specialty American societies and some state medical associations. When the American Board of Family Practice (ABFP) originated in 1969, it incorporated a continuing education requirement as a prerequisite for its original examination for already practicing physicians and for recertification examinations in subsequent years. The 150 hours every three years was accepted as a model by this organization.

Historically, CME endeavors in the United States, which were prompted by the Flexner Report of 1910, have been mostly remedial, attempting to alleviate deficiencies in physicians' medical school or postgraduate medical education. These CME courses were mainly carried out in hospitals, often consisting of technique or cram courses for various techniques and procedures in medicine. The content was not necessarily relevant to the needs of the attending physicians but was controlled by the faculties of these various early postgraduate programs. Often, courses were ineffective in providing new information or knowledge for the doctor to utilize in his practice. Following World War II, the CME emphasis shifted to specialty medical societies and state and county medical societies, which originated numerous programs at their meetings hoping to upgrade the quality of patient care. At the same time, U.S. medical schools began organizing CME departments, implying that students had not finished their medical education merely by graduating from their residency programs. These steps insinuated that physicians should be constant students, adjusting their data base and questing for new knowledge.

The philosophy leading to CME as a requirement was based on the desire of the general practitioner of the 1940s and 1950s to improve patient care as well as his own peer status. Another motive was improvement in hospital privileges. CME thereby began to exert control over the content and quality of various programs. Certainly, the early pioneers in the AAGP did not envision the far-reaching effects of their decision twenty-eight years ago. These early programs did improve the quality of the general practice atmosphere in the United States and were an important factor in developing the new discipline of Family Medicine.

When the American Board of Family Practice was founded in 1969, a definite core content of knowledge and organized continuing education programs, as well as residency programs, was a major ingredient, and the concept of recertification was considered essential to keep the modern family physician in a state of constant learning. No "grandfathers" were to be certified without examination and without documented CME hours. There was also a limited duration of "practice eligibility" incorporated into the American Board of Family Practice (that period will end in 1978). After 1978 the only candidates eligible for the original certifying examination will be those who have finished a residency training program. A one-year grace period was incorporated in the recertification exam in case an individual is unable to sit for the original recertification examination for which he is scheduled. After that year, if he does not sit for or pass the examination he will be dropped from the roles of certified diplomates. He can, however, in subsequent years request and file an application for the recertification procedure, which will be considered by the credentials committee of the ABFP on its merits. A former diplomate in this status who applies for recertification will be required to submit evidence of 300 documented CME hours during the six years prior to his application for recertification.

The recertification procedure consists of four elements:

1. documentation of CME,
2. assessment of licensure status,
3. cognitive examination, and
4. office record review.

CME DOCUMENTATION

All diplomates of the American Board of Family Practice must demonstrate achievement of minimum CME requirements before becoming eligible to sit for the recertification examination (300 hours of acceptable continuing education during the previous six years — an average of 50 hours per year). Documentation can be met by one of the following three types of activities:

1. hours acceptable to the American Academy of Family Physicians for continuing membership in that organization,
2. hours acceptable to the American Medical Association for the Physician's Recognition Award, or
3. the equivalent of hours from either 1 or 2, as approved by the American Board of Family Practice.

Recognizing the many legal ramifications in attempting to establish specific criteria for such a requirement, the procedure is as follows:

Each candidate must certify on the application that he holds unrestricted licensure(s). Such certification will be corroborated. If restricted licensure or absence of licensure is confirmed, the candidate will not be eligible to proceed for the Recertification Procedure.

COGNITIVE EXAMINATION

The cognitive examination in 1977 will be a one-half day written examination primarily covering new advances in the fields applicable to family practice, with special emphasis on knowledge gained in the previous ten years. All candidates for recertification will be expected to maintain a current understanding of new developments and basic knowledge relevant to all the constituent disciplines of family practice (i.e., pediatrics, psychiatry, surgery, internal medicine, community medicine, and obstetrics and gynecology).

The Recertification Cognitive Examination will account for a major portion of the diplomate's score. The fee for this exam will be $150.00. The board will make a serious attempt to provide feedback information to all candidates.

OFFICE RECORD REVIEW

The office record review will be accomplished by asking each diplomate to fill out questionnaires based on his own review of charts for which he bears direct patient care responsibility. There will be ten categories, from which each candidate must choose five. For each of these five categories, he will select four charts, and from each of these charts he will fill out an appropriate questionnaire, reporting whether certain key items of information concerning patient care are contained in the chart. These questionnaires (not the actual charts) will then be mailed to the American Board of Family Practice for evaluation.

A small sample of the candidates, randomly selected, will be asked to submit copies of the original charts from which they completed questionnaires. (Photocopies—not the actual charts—will be sent to preserve the anonymity of the patient, using a numbered identification system.) These charts will be reviewed to determine the validity of the questionnaire procedure, though only a small sample will be asked to send photocopies of the charts from which they filled out their questionnaires. Questionnaires are available for the following categories, from which the candidate will be asked to choose five:

1. Postoperative carcinoma of the breast; mastectomy with or without metastases;

2. coronary artery disease (defined as angina, History of myocardial infarction, or other evidence of coronary insufficiency);
3. depression (adult patient);
4. hypertension (defined as diastolic BP over 100 — adult patient);
5. acute cystitis (adult — male or female);
6. chronic bronchial asthma (adult patient with more than one attack per year);
7. Abnormal vaginal bleeding (adult premenopausal patient);
8. acute duodenal ulcer (adult);
9. diabetes mellitus (adult patient);
10. pediatric patient older than one year who has been followed since birth (current age 1-16 years).

Individuals who cannot meet the office record review requirements of the recertification procedure may submit a written request to the board to take the full two-day certification exam to maintain their diplomate status. The fee for this exam will be $300.00. This option is available only on approval by the board after careful consideration of the candidate's written request, which must contain specific reasons why he cannot provide patient charts to use for the office record review. These reasons will be corroborated by the board. This option is expressly designed for those individuals who wish to maintain certification in family practice but, because of their current professional activities (e.g., emergency room physicians, administrators, military physicians, or educators) cannot meet the requirements of the office record review process as a mechanism to document their actual performance capabilities in family practice.

POSSIBLE FUTURE MEASURES

The original recertification committee considered the possibility of accomplishing a *practice profile* on all diplomates scheduled to sit for recertification. The purpose of this profile was to consider weighting certain elements of the cognitive examination to favor the type of practice in which the individual family physician was engaged. This was found to be impractical, and it was decided to test each candidate across the board. In subsequent years if the practice profile and self-assessment techniques are improved, this could be incorporated into the recertification procedure. Some older physicians who have limited their practice to certain areas of family medicine might favor such a procedure.

There is also an on-going study concerning competency evaluation and proficiency examinations, relating to the actual content of the practicing physician's records and hospital charts. These techniques are not sufficiently refined at the present time, or tested for validity to incorporate them in the present recertification procedure. There is currently a joint project that includes internal medicine, pediatrics, and family practice in a research and development program, in cooperation with the National Board of Medical Examiners, that is attempting to evaluate techniques to study physician competency, especially in the out-patient setting. Certainly, all look forward to the day when one can be confident that the recertification exam will actually verify the status of the practicing diplomate. Early efforts at office chart audits have been subjected to numerous trial runs. Great improvement in the quality of office records has occurred over the last five years due in part to the innovation of problem-oriented medical records, dictation of medical records, and the knowledge by diplomates that their charts will be audited. Many doctors have upgraded their systems. Some have added disease index files to make preparation of the office chart audit easier. At the last survey, over one-half of doctors' records were typed, and the ability to recall pertinent data concerning the specific type disease had markedly improved.

The acceptance of the recertification process by the diplomates of the American Board of Family Practice has been very good. In 1970, there were 1,690 diplomates certified out of almost 2000 tested. It is interesting to note in 1976, when all ABFP diplomates were supposed to be up for recertification, what happened to this original group. Of the 1,690 theoretically eligible, 1,472 (87 percent) have been cleared for the recertification procedure. The remaining 180 break down as follows: 38 diplomates (2.2 percent) have died; 155 have asked to be deferred until 1977 (possibly some of these have retired); and 25 (1.5 percent) gave "no response" after several mailings and are considered unlikely candidates for recertification. This percentage of acceptance by the diplomates is very encouraging.

The mandatory 150 hours every three years of CME requirements of the AAGP evolved over twenty-eight years into a firm basis for the demands of the American Board of Family Practice on their diplomates. This long practice of reporting hours by these physicians alleviates resistance to the board certification and recertification procedure. It has become second nature to those physicians to be involved in continuing medical education.

Chapter 8
Continuing Medical Education: The Role of the State and the Medical Society

Daniel S. Bernstein

Until recently, state legislatures had very little interest in developing legislation involving mandatory continuing education for physicians. The reason for this disinterest is that, traditionally, only licensure was under state control. Moreover, state governments have played little or no role in developing a system that would discipline errant or malpracticing physicians or in understanding the problems of assuring the quality of medical practice. Historically, all that was needed in order to practice medicine or surgery was a medical school diploma and a certificate indicating successful passage of either the state examinations for a medical license or the national medical board examination. Once licensed, the medical practitioner could deliver health care until voluntary retirement. Rarely has a medical license been revoked for malfeasance or malpractice.

A number of events, during the past decade, have motivated state legislatures to develop legislation for mandatory continuing medical education (CME). The reasons for this change are:

1. the passage of Medicare, Medicaid and PSRO legislation by the Federal government;
2. the current malpractice insurance crisis;
3. an increasing public awareness of the "quality" of medical care;
4. medical and subspecialty society pressures for relicensure and recertification; and
5. consumer protection advocacy regarding licensure and relicensure for quality, safety, and competency.

Each of these issues must be considered to understand the actions of state legislatures. The federal role, exemplified by the passage of Title XVIII and XIX (Medicare and Medicaid) and PL 92-603 (PSRO), indicated the federal intent not only to enable the elderly and the poor to receive medical care, but also to assure that the money was spent on health care of the highest "quality." PSRO legislation pursuant to Titles XVIII and XIX, while intending to assure that the monies for health care are equitable and necessary, has emphasized that peer review is the manner in which "quality" will be assured. Under the PSRO legislation continuing medical education programs are to be directed at "deficiencies" in medical care delivery, as determined by medical audit (quality assurance) studies. So far, this has not occurred. Many PSRO supporters have pointed to the lack of funding; much larger amounts of money are needed than are currently appropriated to carry out medical audit studies.

MALPRACTICE AND LICENSURE

The malpractice crisis, on the other hand, has initiated a spate of legislation in a number of states to meet the threat of physician strikes, as physicians in turn face rapidly rising malpractice insurance costs.[1] Most legislation is designed to allow physicians to purchase malpractice insurance at lower rates by spreading the risk through state joint underwriting associations, for state legislators have been made aware that the best punitive action against the malpracticing physician is the state licensing board. In some instances, legislation has been proposed or enacted giving the state board of licensure the power to "discipline" errant physicians. The malpractitioner, defined by R.C. Derbyshire,[2] is "a physician who because of one (or more) of the following factors, causes an injury to his patient, either by commission or ommission, or has the possibility of doing so." These factors are: (1) incompetency, (2) educational obsolescence, (3) carelessness, (4) overworked physicians, (5) greed (more concerned with income than service), and (6) emotional misfit (including alcohol and drug abuse).

Twenty-five states have taken legislative steps to identify the disabled or incompetent physician. These laws generally give to the state board of medical licensure the statutory authority to take disciplinary action against incompetent physicians regardless of the cause of incompetence. The state board of licensure can revoke or suspend the license or can recommend treatment (if ill) or participation in a prescribed program of CME, which could include practicing under medical supervision.

As a possible preventive measure for malpractice, many medical societies have pushed for periodic relicensure, the major requirement for which is demonstrated attendance in CME programs,[3] and some states have passed enabling legislation to ensure that state licensing boards enforce this requirement (Table 8-1). No state licensing board has conducted an outcome study, as of this writing, to demonstrate the possible effectiveness of this requirement. It has been an act of faith that physician attendance in CME will improve or at least maintain high quality medical care delivery. Further, no state licensing board or state medical society has addressed the problem of what should be taught, or who would be the best teachers (generally assumed to be those at medical school teaching centers). Yet, some current programs are taught by those whose background is primarily in basic or clinical research rather than in the common problems of medical care. Are

Table 8-1

MEDICAL RELICENSURE IN THE UNITED STATES

States in which legislation mandates CME as a requirement for relicensure:

1. Michigan—annual relicensure with 50 hours of mandatory CME.
2. New Mexico—triennial relicensure with 120 hours of mandatory CME.

States that are in the planning or implementation stage:

1. Maryland—triennial relicensure in effect; regulations for mandatory CME being rewritten.
2. Kentucky—plans triennial relicensure as of January 1, 1977.
3. Kansas plans triennial relicensure with requirements of 150 hours of mandatory CME beginning July 1, 1978.
4. Ohio—triennial relicensure with requirements of 150 hours of mandatory CME beginning January 1, 1977.
5. Washington—annual relicensure beginning January 1, 1976; option of mandatory CME left to board of licensure (no action taken).
6. Wisconsin—annual relicensure with requirement of 15 hours mandatory CME as of January 1, 1978.
7. Massachusetts—biennial relicensure as of January 1, 1976; no mandatory CME requirements.
8. Oregon—no relicensure; medical society requires 50 hours CME for membership yearly.

they, necessarily, the "best" teachers for improving the quality of medical practice?

Some specialty medical societies have begun to develop a rationale for recertification. The American Board of Internal Medicine has developed and implemented a voluntary recertification exam; the American Board of Surgery has one in process. Claude Welch articulated his own position, which probably reflects a majority one for surgeons.[4] He notes several ways recertification could be accomplished: written reexamination, individual participation in a variety of education activities, or a peer review system akin to that projected by full PSRO implementation (a surgeon's operative record would be considered as the basis for recertification). Other specialty societies have varying requirements utilizing CME as a basis for recertification. None has lobbied or initiated attempts for state or federal legislation regarding mandatory recertification or relicensure.

The American health consumer has had an increasing awareness of health problems and an increasing level of expectation as to the quality of health care delivery. This has occurred as the image of the physician has changed, which is probably attributable to the increase in communications. The physician has often been depicted as wealthy, not compassionate, and sometimes not even up to date. Advances in medical technology and treatment are reported in the press almost instantaneously and before adequate medical substantiation which, unfortunately, raises public expectation. Legislators, both state and federal, upset over spiraling health costs and the enormous investments in research over the past twenty-five years, have a scanty knowledge of real medical accomplishments in health care delivery. In other words, the medical profession has suffered from a lack of a public relations effort to relate the large investments in research to the innovations and advances in medical care delivery, thus rationalizing these expenditures.

PUBLIC POLICY CONCERNS

The public and its elected legislators have shown an increased medical awareness and have heightened their demands for cost accountability, physician competency, and an efficient means for assuring the safety of medical care delivery. The existing situation indicates that if the PSROs do not function to the satisfaction of the federal and state governments, these legislative bodies will pass laws which would have third party review of medical care. These laws would mandate punitive measures that could damage the physician-patient relationship and alter the medical care delivery system drastically. PSROs probably represent a last chance for the profession to monitor its own affairs. Failure of the PSROs augurs dire consequences.

There are a number of public policy issues concerned with (1) the role of CME as a requirement for relicensure; (2) the role of the federal and state governments and the medical societies, provided CME demonstrates a positive effect in maintaining or increasing the quality of health care delivery; and (3) quality assurance of medical care delivery to the public.

In terms of utilizing CME as a means for recertification or relicensure, the medical consensus appears to be that CME is a viable instrument in the process.[5,6] Evaluation of this concept has not been attempted, but it is reasonable to assume that a large percentage of physicians would attend CME courses if relicensure or recertification were a necessity to maintain licensure or specialty certification. Also, the larger percentage of physicians attend CME programs because of their own desire to be current and to deliver the best care to their patients. However, the only useful assessment of individual (or group) quality of care delivery is by outcome measurements. Furthermore, outcome measurements can only be measured against defined criteria of quality care, assessment of deficiencies, and a method for correction of the deficiencies. Such correction is assumed to result from CME, medical consultation by "experts," and other teaching exercises.

RECOMMENDATIONS

1. That the federal government establish a *separately* funded program, carried out by each of the 203 PSROs, for training PSRO personnel in methods of *medical audit* to outline deficiencies in medical care. These programs would also focus on developing local *consortia* under PSRO auspices for corrective education designed to meet the elaborated deficiencies. Consortia can be construed as groups of medical educators from medical schools, teaching hospitals, specialty medical societies, universities, and other teaching institutions.

2. That the federal government, under the Bureau of Quality Assurance, fund a program which would evaluate the impact of CME on medical practice. This program would involve every PSRO and would utilize individual and group data to provide regional norms for medical care delivery.

3. That relicensure in individual states would depend on PSRO certification of physician practice and performance. It is recognized that this recommendation would place an enormous burden on the PSROs;

but it has the effect that physicians, through a process of peer review, would be able to distinguish those physicians whose practice was nonconforming.

4. That each state would, through legislation, empower the board of registration and discipline to deny relicensure to any physician identified by the PSRO as one who does not meet PSRO standards of practice. This would bypass the difficulty of physicians "disciplining" other physicians.

CONCLUSION

The current practice in those states where relicensure is based on attendance in CME courses has little to recommend its continuance. If the above recommendations were adopted, a process of objective evaluation of physician practice and the effect of CME on it would be instituted.

The public assurance of quality medical care is a different and difficult issue. The public has representation on the boards of each PSRO, and, in a few states, nonprofessionals participate on boards of medical licensure. It would not serve the public or the profession well to indicate publicly those physicians whose practice is allegedly nonconforming or incompetent until the time comes when the state board will refuse renewal or will suspend the license. The damage to a physician so accused of incompetence by the publicizing of his or her "trial" *before* action by the state board of licensure would be irreparable, especially if the physician were innocent. But should such practices come to the license procedure, full disclosure of the reasons for denial of license will be public information.

It is recognized that the cost of implementing these recommendations is immense, but still in proportion to total health costs (which in 1976 will certainly exceed $120 billion). Industry generally allows 1 percent of total revenues to maintain quality control. It is estimated that $500 million spent in fully implementing PSROs would probably contain the spiraling costs of health care while providing quality assurance. This would mean an investment of less than one-half of one percent to assure quality health expenditures.

NOTES

1. W.H.L. Dornette, "Role of the Healing Arts Licensing Board in

the Current Medical Malpractice Crisis," presented at the annual meeting of State Licensing Boards, Chicago, Illinois, January 30, 1976.

2. R. C. Derbyshire, "Relicensure—1975," presented at the annual meeting of State Licensing Boards, Chicago, Illinois, January 30, 1976.

3. W. H. L. Dornette, "Ohio Strives to Resolve Malpractice Problem," *Journal of Legal Medicine* 4 (January 1976): 30-32.

4. C. E. Welch, "Quality Care, Quasi-Care, and Quackery," Bulletin of the American College of Surgeons 58 (November 1973): 7-12.

5. J. S. Millis, "The Impact of Relicensure Upon Postgraduate Medical Education," *Modern Medicine* 38 (June 1970): 86-89.

6. M. Pennington, "A Review of Mandatory Continuing Medical Education in Oregon," *Western Journal of Medicine* 120 (January 1974): 80-87.

Part III
Evaluation of CME Programs

Chapter 9
The Impact of CME on the Quality of Care: What are the Results?

Osler Peterson

Continuing medical education is usually undertaken for one of the following reasons: as a repair job, to remedy failures of medical education and clinical training; to bring new knowledge to the physician; or to support the quality of medical care. The innumerable lectures that have been given on the judicious use of antibiotics and other drugs are examples of this last genre.

There are two commonly held propositions about CME. The first states that physicians who need it most obtain it least; and the second states that it is the older doctor who needs CME, the assumption being that the young, recently graduated physician knows what he needs to conduct a competent practice. Both positions, one suspects, contain some truth.

GENERAL PRACTITIONERS AND CME

This author first became deeply acquainted with CME while doing an in-depth study of general practitioners, which included detailed records of the continuing education habits of the practitioners.[1] There was a variation in the amount of time individual GPs had devoted to continuing education in the previous year. Some had, for all practical purposes, no exposure to continuing education; others had attended the equivalent of two to three weeks of postgraduate education, as judged from the number and duration of meetings attended.

There was no association between the amount of their continuing medical education efforts and an adjudged quality of practice, nor was greater interest in CME characteristic of the better physicians. The aphorism that the doctors who do not need continuing education get the most and those most in need of education get the least was not true for this group.

At the conclusion of this study of general practice, there was a further investigation that has not been published. In this second study internal medicine practices were first examined to ascertain whether they were generally similar to general practices.[2] Aside from the fact that internists treated few children and practiced no obstetrics, their work was very much like general practice. Internal medicine was characterized by a wide spectrum of disease problems. Care was comprehensive and normally continuous. Because of the different patient age structures in general practice and internal medicine, the disease patterns tended to be somewhat different — more acute diseases in the former and more chronic disease in the latter. When the determination had been made that there were more similarities than differences, a sample of internists was drawn and studied.

The specific purpose of the internist study was to determine if a major conclusion of the first investigation could be verified. This conclusion was that the quality of care given by general practitioners was directly related to the amount of their clinical training in internal medicine. Our hypothesis is represented by Figure 9-1, which shows what is essentially a learning curve. We assumed that general practitioners whose clinical training was normally short would be found on the left and lower portion of this curve. The internists, whose training is normally longer, were expected to cluster on the higher portions of the quality curve on the right of the graph.

That hypothesis was approximately true. The reality is demonstrated in Figure 9-2. The general practitioners who had short and generally poor training were indeed clustered on the lower part of the curve, and the internists with generally longer training were concentrated on the higher part of the curve. However, where their clinical training overlapped, the differences were significant statistically — the result was unlikely to be related to a chance occurrence. These different reactions to clinical training suggest that we are dealing with two different subpopulations. It is well to recall that this study was done from 1953-1955. The type of people who gained admission to medical schools prior to those years and ended up in general practice are probably not now admitted to medical school. The increasing number of candidates for medical school has probably skewed the selection more toward students with the characteristics of specialists, and specifically the internists.

In addition to the significant differences in the quality of clinical care given, there was a second observation of similar importance. The

Figure 9-1

LEARNING CURVE (HYPOTHESIS)

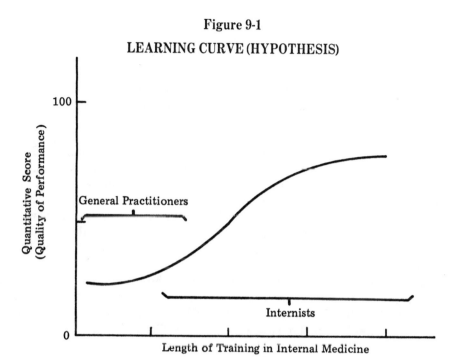

Figure 9-2

LEARNING CURVE (REALITY)

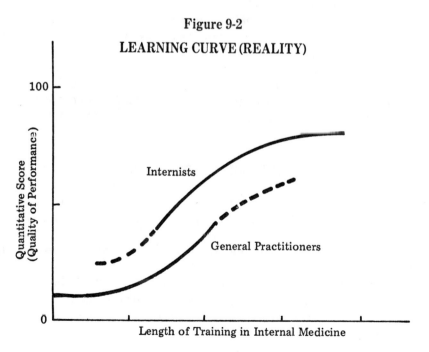

quality of general practice deteriorated after a few years of practice. Among the internists, on the other hand, there was no evidence of loss of skill up to age 65, the cutoff point. In other words, the longer clinical training of the internists seemed to result in more durable knowledge and skills. Internists seemed to be a homogeneous group with respect to quality of medical care, and no association with CME was expected or found.

The internists' study habits were different from those of general practitioners. The latter normally went to meetings and courses. The internists naturally attended the clinical meetings such as sessions of the American College of Physicians, but they also seemed frequently to arrange their own education. An example was an internist who had scheduled a week or two with Dr. Frank Wilson at the University of Michigan to learn vectorcardiography. Internists in general seemed to be well read, and their need for education was much less than in the case of the general practitioners. The products of medical education have changed. The general practitioner at whom so much continuing education was normally directed is now a small group. He is being replaced by a family doctor whose clinical training is better and whose practice is likely to include a team approach. These characteristics provide considerable assurance about the quality of his care.

The family doctors — internists, pediatricians, or family practitioners — who have largely replaced the general practitioner certainly do not need the "repair work" that was lavished on the latter. Yet, the veneration of new knowledge has not abated. Medical education directed at keeping the doctors current is still important. Education designed to support the quality of medical care probably can now be provided with somewhat greater success than was possible when practitioners were dichotomized in clinically well-trained specialty groups and minimally trained general practitioner groups.

PROFESSIONALIZING CME

Another important change is the professionalization of CME. As a clinical fellow at the Thorndike Laboratory, this author often lectured on infectious diseases at New England hospitals to audiences of mainly general practitioners. Planning was very casual, and one wonders if the young resident who received the fee was not the main beneficiary of the exercise. The process of professionalization which began with the appointment of full-time directors of medical education has been given much greater rigor by Clement Brown's Bi-Cycle concept and John Williamsons' "Achievable Benefits Not Achieved" measure.[3,4]

This greater rigor is an important and necessary step for effective educational programs but is probably not sufficient.

During recent years one has observed that directors of medical education have been increasingly included in hospital administration. Their titles would suggest a certain amount of authority and influence—Director of Medical Services, Vice President for Medical Affairs, and the like. This step is critical.

It is not necessary to describe again the educational system established by the Northern California Kaiser Medical Group, but some of the central features that illustrate the importance of imbedding educational programs in the medical organization should be mentioned. The first step in the Northern California Kaiser quality program is to locate evidence of unsatisfactory quality. One then asks if the quality defect is important enough to receive attention, and if so, how will it be handled and who will be responsible—all organizational questions. The doctors who join the Kaiser organizations presumably accept the constraints imposed by a group, so they probably represent a fertile soil for quality improving measures.

The community hospital, a more typical example of a medical care institution concerned with the quality of patient care, is a collection of individuals with different and varying competencies and goals. Therefore, the problems of patient care quality and the possible effectiveness of CME are different from those in a prepaid group practice. Some hospitals are coping with their quality problems and others are not. Those with full-time directors of medical education (DMEs) fully supported by the trustees are probably a select group that cleave to a higher standard of care than those without DMEs or formal educational programs. It is unlikely, however, that there is the same degree of agreement on need for education and quality standards in hospitals as is found in the generally more cohesive group practices. Hospitals that effectively monitor and enforce a high quality of patient care are still a relatively small minority.

The importance of embedding the continuing education process in the hospital organization is worth heavy emphasis. Though there are many clinical studies of treatment effectiveness, information on how adequately effective clinical processes are utilized in individual institutions is quite limited. Since it would be unethical to randomize patients into "good" or "bad" hospitals, evidence on the relationship between organization and quality will always have to be limited to observational studies, and there are several examples that point to a close correlation between good organization and good outcomes.

Figure 9-3 shows the survival rate of all patients treated for carcinoma of the cervix in upstate New York during one year.[5] The top line, which represents the survival of patients treated at Roswell Park Memorial Hospital, a specialized institution for cancer patients, is clearly the best. The second line shows the survival of patients treated in teaching hospitals, and the third line shows the survival of patients treated in other hospitals of these same cities—Rochester, Albany, Syracuse, and Buffalo. The final line represents the survival of patients treated outside these metropolitan centers. The result of treatment of cervical cancer is greatly influenced by the stage of the disease when treatment begins, so the authors have stratified patients as "early" or "late." The patients treated at Roswell Park included fewer stage I cancers (42 percent and 39 percent in the two study

Figure 9-3

TEN-YEAR SURVIVAL RATE IN CANCER OF THE CERVIX,
STAGES I-IV, BASED ON PATIENTS TREATED IN 1949

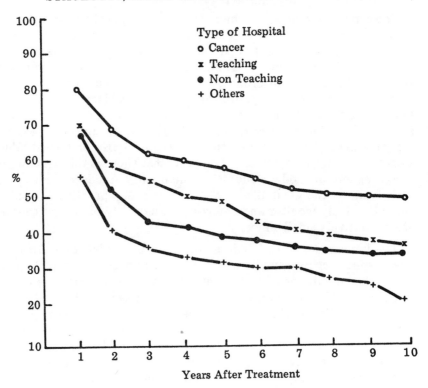

years) than the other hospitals. The community hospitals, which had the poorest survival rates, treated more patients with Stage I cancers (68 percent in both years) than any other. The authors attributed better results obtained by Roswell Park to (1) the much greater experience of physicians, (2) the variety of specialists (a team including gynecologists, surgeons, radiotherapists, radiation physicists, radiation technicians), and (3) facilities that allow optimum treatment to be given to more patients. It was also noted that there were substantial variations in end results of different teaching hospitals. One service directed by a gynecologist with a special interest in this cancer had more patients and achieved better results than other teaching hospitals. This study also says something about how specialized services should be organized, both internally and regionally.

There is another organizational point to be made. Roswell Park physicians treated 127 and 156 patients in the two study years. The teaching hospitals with the second best outcomes treated 15 to 37 people. The small community hospital averaged about 3.5 patients per hospital year. (For the last group, experience was clearly insufficient to provide a base for expertise.) Roswell Park, which had, on the average, more than one patient weekly to treat had a much better experience base on which to build up treatment skills and quality of care.

OTHER CME STUDIES

Table 9-1, adapted from Yankauer, shows neonatal mortality in hospitals of upstate New York by type and number of deliveries.[6] In this study Yankauer calculated birth weight-adjusted death rates to account for this major risk variable. As the table makes clear, the death rate falls as the experience of the hospital increases. The death rate is also lower in hospitals with more teaching responsibility. An institution with both pediatric and obstetric clinical training programs had a somewhat better outcome than hospitals with only one of the programs. If this association is accepted as cause and effect rather than a result of patient selection, one must recognize that the effects of education are difficult to separate from the effects of organization. The important organizational details, which include staffing, structure, and goals, probably increase in step with educational responsibilities.

The next example is in many ways the most interesting. The surgeons at the University Department of Surgery of the General Infirmary at Leeds (England) have been doing clinical trials for several years.[7] One member of the group, deDombal, also studied cost benefits and clinical decision processes. In the study considered here he com-

Table 9-1

NEONATAL MORTALITY, ADJUSTED FOR BIRTH WEIGHT,
BY HOSPITAL OF BIRTH

No. of Births per Annum	Birth Weight Adjusted for Death Rate
>100	18.7
100-499	19.0
500-599	17.4
1000 or more	16.9
Number of approved interns or residents	17.6
Approved residents for OB only	17.4
Approved residents for OB and pediatrics	16.0

pared the accuracy of computer versus surgeons' diagnoses. The patient population was made up of those who came to the hospital with acute abdominal pain. In comparing the accuracy of diagnoses of various doctors, some interesting trends were shown. The admitting diagnosis, presumably made by a casualty officer who had no responsibility for the patient's treatment and might not have had all available information, was quite inaccurate (45 percent correct). The house surgeons (junior members of the surgical team) were more accurate (72 percent correct). The registrars (who normally have had two to eight years or more surgical experience) achieved an accuracy of 77 percent, and the senior clinicians, the most experienced, achieved a rate of nearly 80 percent. Interestingly, the computer diagnostic system utilization of the same data as the clinicians used achieved an accuracy of over 90 percent.

During the course of the experiment, the feedback of computer diagnostic information was described as follows:

> We did not at once inform members of the clinical team of the computer's predictions, but we did discuss the case with them once this initial decision and management had been made and undertaken. Certainly after each "take-in" day we spent some time discussing the relevant cases with members of the clinical team, providing them with a delayed form of "feedback" and analysis of their own and the computer-aided system's performance.

Figure 9-4

PERCENT OF PATIENTS WITH PERFORATED APPENDIX AT OPERATION BY STAGE OF TRIAL[7]

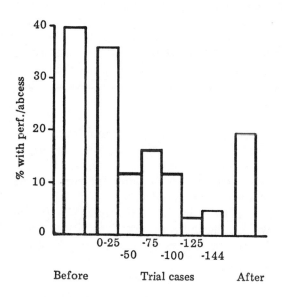

Figure 9-4 demonstrates what happened to the proportion of patients with a diagnosis of acute appendicitis who also had perforations at the time of operation during the period when the surgeons were being tested against the computer. Before the study 40 percent had this complication, but the percentage declined in an irregular fashion down to about 4 or 5 percent toward the conclusion of the study period. Interestingly, it then bounced up to about 20 percent in the period immediately after the cessation of the study.

One of the diagnostic categories used was nonspecific abdominal pain, which the authors agreed was not a diagnosis, but nonetheless a necessary category. In Figure 9-5 the proportion of patients with this diagnosis who came to the operation but had a "negative" laparotomy is shown. Before the study approximately a quarter of patients in this category had a negative laparotomy. As in the case of a perforated appendix, however, this proportion dropped during the study and rebounded sharply after its conclusion. DeDombal surmises the possible effect of the experiment as follows:

But equally it would be idle to ignore the possibility that the discipline forced on our clinical colleagues, the constraint of collecting clinical information to complete a form containing a series of rigidly defined patient attributes, the constant emphasis on the reliability of clinical data collected, and the rapid "feed-back" from the computer-aided system may have combined to account for at least part of the improvement seen during our survey. Sadly, it seems that the effect was short-lived, in that once the trial was over the clinicians' performances reverted to something like their previous level....

DeDombal did not title this a "Hawthorne effect," though this clearly was what he described. The participants in the original Hawthorne study explained their productivity decline at the experiments' termination by saying that former participants were no longer interested. Apparently, the surgeons reacted similarly.

It is not easy to institutionalize or routinize the type of organized activity that provoked the increased productivity in the Hawthorne experiment or the greater accuracy in deDombal's study. This is why

Figure 9-5

PERCENT OF PATIENTS WITH NONSPECIFIC ABDOMINAL PAIN WITH NEGATIVE LAPAROTOMY BY STAGE OF TRIAL[7]

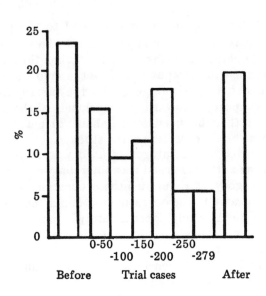

good managers are paid so well. DeDombal's experimental method bore about the same relationship to surgical care as a good tutor's relation to a student and probably could not be easily or widely replicated at reasonable costs. It should be recognized that a "Hawthorne effect" was probably also involved in Clement Brown's experiments.

Another example also involves perinatal death rates (there are enough deaths to make this type of study practical).[8] In this study the better results obtained in a prepaid group practice were attributed to a monitoring system that brought every infant death to early attention. Clearly if quality is to be maintained, someone must be aware of what quality is. A second variable was the group's selection of obstetricians which was thorough and exacting. These are also characteristics of good organization.

THE EXAMPLE OF FLORENCE NIGHTINGALE

Since the real purpose of education is to maintain or elevate the quality of care, it will be useful to recall the experience of Florence Nightingale in improving the British army's medical services, because she understood the several issues involved.[9] When Miss Nightingale and her nurses arrived at Scutari in Turkey, she found the conditions in the military hospital abominable. The soldiers who were wounded in the fighting were brought across the Black Sea from Russia by ship, where the death rate was quite low. That state of affairs was reversed after reaching the hospital.

Miss Nightingale noted that hospital deaths were due to "zymotic diseases such as scurvy, enteric fever, cholera, diarrhea, and dysentery," not directly to wounds. She saw and understood the association between the number of patients in the hospital, overcrowding, and the mortality rate. Her sanitary improvements included 5,114 "hand carts or large basketfuls of filth removed, flushing out stopped up sewers and latrines 466 times, the burial of 35 carcasses of animals found in and about the hospitals, washing of bed sheets and shirts, and replacing unclean clothes which the soldiers had been wearing since they left the battlefield." She explained the excessive mortality by "frightful overcrowding and want of ventilation, draining, cleanliness, and hospital comforts." Her work at Scutari followed John Snow's discovery of the transmission of cholera through drinking water by some five years, and she was almost certainly aware of it.[10]

Miss Nightingale was, above all else, a tough, realistic and farsighted woman who understood well the uses of power. She soon realized after returning to England to a hero's welcome that, dramatic as her work in the Crimea had been, it was not enough. She therefore set to work to reform the British army's medical services, where she met great resistance. She succeeded only after years of effort and frequent use of statistics at least as dramatic as the Scutari death rates.

CONCLUSIONS

If the quality of care is to be improved in this country, several changes will have to be made. First, we must list the organizations whose quality of care *is* good: likely including teaching hospitals, major group practices, and some nonuniversity hospitals with full-time staff. These are institutions in which there is an organization whose chief business is to monitor care and assure that it is of high quality, while recognizing and correcting unsatisfactory care. However, an organization by itself cannot solve all problems. It is necessary to have a manpower policy that assures an appropriate relationship between the number of specialists in surgery, cardiology, psychiatry, or family practice and the need for their services. Large numbers of trained surgeons with exceedingly small work loads are a symptom of excess supply, which probably has important implications for quality of care.[11] Just as the manpower supply must be adjusted to the needs of the population, so must facilities be planned in relation to these needs. The great excess of coronary care units, to cite a common example, has caused a situation where some have too few patients to keep the unit team in practice.[12] In the case of radiation therapy, the proper model is Roswell Park, not the local community hospital.[13]

Throughout this chapter reference has been made to the fact that CME now operates under serious handicaps. When these major organizational changes have taken place, as is likely following enactment of national health insurance, CME should be far more effective because it will be an accepted part of the service organizations rather than an "add-on" or an extension service from a remote university hospital. Under these circumstances, CME will operate under conditions more commensurate with its potential.

NOTES

1. O. L. Peterson *et al.,* "An Analytical Study of North Carolina

General Practice," *The Journal of Medical Education* 31, Part 2 (December 1956).

2. R. S. Spain *et al.*, "The Quality of Patient Care Given by Internists" (unpublished), available from Dr. Peterson, Harvard School of Public Health.

3. C. R. Brown, Jr., and D. S. Fleisher, "The Bi-Cycle Concept — Relating Continuing Education Directly to Patient Care," *New England Journal of Medicine* 284, Supplement (May 20, 1971).

4. J. W. Williamson, M. Alexander, and G. E. Miller, "Continuing Education and Patient Care Research," *JAMA* 201, no.12 (September 18, 1967): 118-122.

5. J. B. Graham and F. P. Paloucek, "Where Should Cancer of the Cervix Be Treated? A Preliminary Report," *American Journal of Obstetrics and Gynecology* 87 (October 1, 1963): 405-409.

6. A. Yankauer and N. C. Allaway, "An Analysis of Hospital Neonatal Mortality Rates in New York State," *AMA Journal of Diseases of Children* 95 (1958): 240-244.

7. F. T. deDombal *et al.*, "Human and Computer-Aided Diagnosis of Abdominal Pain: Further Report with Emphasis on Performance of Clinicians," *British Medical Journal* 1 (March 2, 1974): 376-380.

8. S. Shapiro, L. Weiner, and P. M. Densen, "Comparison of Prematurity and Perinatal Mortality in a General Population and in the Population of a Prepaid Group Practice, Medical Care Plan," *American Journal of Public Health* 48 (1958): 170-187.

9. Florence Nightingale, *Notes on Matters Affecting the Health, Efficiency and Hospital Administration of the Birtish Army, Founded Chiefly on the Experience of the Late War* (London: Harrison & Sons, 1858); available Houghton Library, Harvard University.

10. B. W. Richardson and Wade Hampton Frost, *Snow on Cholera* (New York: Commonwealth Fund, 1936).

11. *Surgery in the United States. A Summary Report of the Study on Surgical Services for the United States* (Baltimore: Lewis Advertising Co., 1975), pp. 21-98.

12. B. S. Bloom and O. L. Peterson, "Patient Needs and Medical-Care Planning. The Coronary-Care Unit as a Model," *New England Journal of Medicine* 290 (May 23, 1974): 1171-1177.

13. B. S. Bloom, O. L. Peterson, and S. P. Martin, "Radiation Therapy in New Hampshire, Massachusetts and Rhode Island — Output and Cost," *New England Journal of Medicine* 286 (January 27, 1972): 189-194.

Chapter 10
Evaluating the Evaluators of Continuing Medical Education Programs

Sol Levine

Anyone who approaches the literature on continuing medical education has to be impressed with the wide range of concerns and the diverse expectations that lie behind this effort. Continuing medical education is often viewed as a major means of overcoming the deficiencies or incompetencies of a small proportion of physicians (5 percent is the conventional assumption). At other times, CME is regarded as an indispensable mechanism by which the average physician can keep up with the tremendous growth of medical scientific knowledge. Advocates of CME argue that medical training must continue after medical school so the adult physician is not rendered obsolete by the rapid developments in medical science. These persons say the physician must be informed of the latest developments in the medical armamentarium and must adopt desirable medical innovations. Conversely, CME is deemed to be important for the physician to avoid inappropriate medical intervention that could produce iatrogenic illness. Some advocates see CME as another major means of controlling the spiraling costs of health care by minimizing unnecessary procedures and hospital admissions. Some go so far as to view it as a major mechanism for improving the health care delivery system.

The CME literature is characterized by considerable disagreement. Writers and evaluators of CME range from those who are sanguine about its potential (some even urge it to be a standard and required practice for medical recertification) to those who view it as superfluous, ineffective, excessively costly, and unnecessarily burdensome. The literature also ranges widely in the evidence used to support various assertions.

Rarely does one encounter a systematic and rigorous evaluation study of continuing medical education. Occasionally, some critics present empirical data; more often, the supporting data are derived from secondary sources, i.e., the findings of other investigators. Most of the articles consist of various commentaries, deliberations or overall assessments. This chapter is in keeping with most of the literature in the field in that it is not based on a systematic study; it does not present new empirical data. The purpose of this chapter is to attempt a judicious and critical overview of the assessments and evaluations of others and to place them in a proper perspective.

TRADITIONAL CME

One conspicuous feature of CME, especially in its earlier history, is its commitment to the assumption that the successful transmission of new information or skills to the physician is a worthwhile end in and of itself. In addition, one often encounters a related and accompanying assumption that the transmission of new information will lead to behavior change and, consequently, to beneficial effects on health care. Those who subscribe to these assumptions tend to focus their attention on how well the various types of information and skills are transmitted and retained over time, as well as the relative efficacy of different media techniques and other aspects of instruction. A number of CME studies report on such features as the characteristics of those who attend and the frequency of attendance. However, there has been a dearth of information on CME's effectiveness in terms of hard criteria variables such as the behavior of the physician or the end quality of medical care.

Critics of what may be called traditional continuing medical education do not deny that it is desirable to impart new information and skills to physicians as well as to other health personnel. They do question, however, whether traditional CME methods are effective even in terms of the limited criteria by which most advocates would judge their success. Even more, they find little evidence to support the notion that participation in continuing education courses leads to changes in physician behavior. They explicitly challenge the assumption that there is any relationship between exposure to traditional CME courses and the improvement of the recipient population. Finally, critics raise the inevitable question of whether the relative time, energies, and monies devoted to CME could not be spent more fruitfully on other types of inputs into the health system.

Those who express reservations about traditional CME's effectiveness have been confronted with little data to challenge their skepticism. As Lewis and Hassanein state: ". . . it is disturbing to note the lack of evidence that current efforts are worth the time and energy being expended."[1] These same authors produced one of the most extensive searches of the literature in the field. They point out that all kinds of administrative statistics have been compiled that are essentially descriptive and bear little on the effectiveness of the teaching endeavor. Data have tended to reflect more the operation of the programs, not their objectives, achievements, or end products. These same authors also characterize a number of other studies as little more than "marketing research" — studies that have been concerned largely with the needs, attitudes, and interests of physicians who have participated in CME programs. While the authors grant that it is important to know these operational features of continuing medical education, they emphasize the need to ascertain whether their programs do, in fact, change the behavior of participants. In short, most of the studies of traditional CME efforts have been of little value because they have had methodological deficiencies or have lacked hard measures of outcome.

Lewis and Hassanein also examined studies that were more concerned with changes in behavior effected by continuing medical education. Although these studies, too, have methodological deficiencies, they have tended almost uniformly to yield negative results. One is reminded, for example, that O.L. Peterson, who carried out the now classic study of practitioners in North Carolina, also found no evidence that participation in CME affected the quality of care rendered by physicians.

They also report on a study by J.G. Roney and G.M. Roark, who obtained the cooperation of a small percentage of physicians in Kansas to participate in a CME study. Those investigators found no evidence that there was any change in the patterns of practice among those who participated in the program. While the limits of the study design and the scope of the research effort are recognized, their findings, together with those of other investigators, appear to throw further doubt on the potential impact of CME. Lewis and Hassanein also report their own study of 57 percent of 2,090 physicians in Kansas who participated in CME programs at some time from 1956 to 1965. They report that maternal and obstetrical death rates in various regions were not related to the degree of participation by local physicians in CME courses in obstetrics and pediatrics.

The total picture that emerges, then, is that there is little hard data to endorse traditional continuing medical education. One might be tempted to take a cynical stance and view CME as further testimony to the inveterate American faith in the value of education and in the belief that "activity," especially when it is a learning activity, is worthwhile. Traditional CME could also be faulted for its "rationalistic" bias in its commitment to achieving change in behavior through the mere transmission of information.

Despite the apparent lack of success of traditional CME programs, one must be careful and circumspect about potential implications. It would be wrong to assume that because CME, *as it has been practiced*, has not demonstrated success, the concept should thus be readily rejected. Indeed, as one examines its major features, it is not surprising that the results have been overwhelmingly negative. First, the input of the variable has been weak. For the most part physicians who have participated in the program have been exposed to relatively brief instruction (in many cases, just a few hours). Second, in accordance with past conventional practice, physicians have elected to attend or not to attend different instructional sessions depending on their preferences or inclinations. Popular wisdom informs us that physicians, as other professionals, attend conferences for many reasons besides that of acquiring knowledge. Indeed, for many conference participants the acquisition of new information might not be the salient concern. Third, the material traditionally presented and treated at CME sessions has not necessarily been geared to meeting the felt needs of the participants. Fourth, whatever information the physician might acquire has not been rewarded or reinforced subsequently.

A real test of the efficacy of CME would be found in the evaluation of a program that has met and overcome these past limitations. Can continuing medical education be effective if the input is more intensive, longer, and more sustained; if the felt needs of physicians are addressed; if the acquired material is reinforced subsequently; in short, if the knowledge imparted is a much more powerful variable or input?

RECENT TRENDS IN CME

Traditional continuing medical education should be distinguished from the more recent and emerging developments in the field. Three main new trends in continuing medical education are specified in a study by G.H. Escovitz:[2]

First, responsibility for continuing medical education has begun to shift toward the community hospital. Second, self-evaluation is being used as a stimulus to learning. Third, concern for relating education efforts to the analysis of the quality of patient care has increased. These three trends are mutually supportive in many ways.

The effort to relate CME to evaluation of the quality of medical care is a significant development. For CME to contribute to the quality of medical care, Escovitz sees four logical steps which must be taken: "(1) setting standards for care, (2) comparing actual performance to standards, (3) planning and implementing 'remedial' programs when necessary, and (4) evaluating the extent to which the first three steps have resulted in the desired change in patient care."[3]

Clearly, CME is being formulated and designed in the present period to attempt to free itself from its past deficiencies and to provide more relevancy, more "teeth," and more leverage. One of the major leaders in this development is Clement R. Brown, who has been critical of traditional CME practices still in use. Brown deplores the fact that most CME has failed to relate learning to patient care needs. He feels the relationship can be established by[4]

> two newly developed methodologies: (1) by the identification of specific deficiencies in patient care in the hospital setting combined with programs for correction; (2) by the establishment of a communications network for consultation on a patient-care problem between family physician or the community specialist and appropriate specialist at the university or regional medical center.

Leaning on the work of Williamson, Brown and his colleagues have developed a "Bi-Cycle" approach, which they report has been employed successfully at Chestnut Hill Hospital (see Chapter 2). Brown and his associates summon various data to demonstrate the success of their programs, though they acknowledge they have had failures as well. They decry the movement toward compulsory attendance at traditional CME programs and argue that the kind of experimental programs they have developed should be acknowledged and accredited. "Such participative, self-help, problem-solving, need meeting, patient care, improving educational systems warrant the support of accrediting or certifying agencies now."[5]

Brown's stance toward traditional medical education has been echoed and affirmed by Escovitz, who has developed his own modified version of the Bi-Cycle approach. Like Brown, Escovitz sees CME constructed around demonstrated problems in providing patient care, the establishment of appropriate criteria or standards of good quality care, and the development of consensus regarding these standards. Escovitz emphasizes the need to involve the physicians who provide the clinical care. He also believes that the deliberations, discussions, and disagreements which occur in the process are an important part of the learning process. A series of steps occur in which actual performance is compared with the criteria established; then appropriate remedial instruction is indicated. Again, data can be acquired to assess the input of remedial instruction on performance.

Escovitz makes one *crucial* observation. In many cases, poor quality of care is not a function of physician ignorance but stems from administrative, organizational, or sociological factors.

There is little question that the critics of traditional CME present a formidable argument. The new approach that they propose is more in accord with what we know about the conditions under which learning takes place and how behavior is modified. The fact that increasing numbers of physicians practice medical care in organizational settings also attests to the importance of carrying out CME in relevant organizational contexts.

However, before one becomes overly committed to CME in its more modern cloak, one must raise a number of questions to subject the newer CME programs to similar critical scrutiny. How well does the modern approach work in different organizational settings? What are the costs as well as the gains in terms of such variables as money, time, caseload, and personnel retention? Does physician determination of good quality of care correspond to the definition that patients would employ? For example, to what extent are such factors as waiting, scheduling, and patient education considered in establishing standards of quality of care? What organizational preconditions must exist before physicians are willing to submit to and cooperate with new forms of CME? What kinds of incentives and sanctions are necessary?

Indeed, it may be asked whether one cannot achieve some CME objectives by setting explicit organizational objectives, by establishing appropriate organizational rewards and sanctions, and by the introduction of evaluation forms. In fact, one should enquire to what extent new CME methods have worked because of the existence of organizational incentives and sanctions, independent of the instructional mechanisms used? Conversely, would continuing medical education work without these incentives or sanctions?

Although the improvement of the delivery system requires mechanisms that go far beyond continuing medical education, it is possible for CME to make a significant contribution. To what extent this contribution can be made under different conditions requires systematic, rigorous, and refined evaluation studies, which thus far have not been characteristic of the field.

NOTES

1. C.E. Lewis, M.D. and R.S. Hassanein, "Continuing Medical Education — An Epidemiological Evaluation," *New England Journal of Medicine* 282 (January 29, 1970): 254.

2. G.H. Escovitz, M.D., "Continuing Education and Quality of Care," *The Hospital Medical Staff* (March 1974): 23.

3. Ibid., p. 30.

4. C.R. Brown, M.D., and H.S.M. Uhl, "Mandatory Continuing Education: Sense or Nonsense?" *JAMA* 213 (September 7, 1970): 1662.

5. Ibid., p. 1667.

Chapter 11
The Role of PSROs in Conducting and Evaluating Continuing Medical Education Programs

Alan R. Nelson

The portions of PL 92-603 that establish Professional Standards Review Organizations are very specific in assigning to PSROs the responsibility for assuring that services provided under Titles V, XVIII, and XIX are medically necessary and of reasonable quality. The review for appropriate utilization of services is technically easy, and most PSROs have, at least, a functioning and organized operation to conduct utilization review. Individual PSROs and the PSRO program in general are now beginning to ask more seriously what is meant by quality assurance and how is quality assurance carried out.

QUALITY ASSURANCE

Quality assurance can be achieved in one of two ways:

1. The services being rendered to eligible recipients can be reviowed by one or more peers if these services fail to meet the basic screening criteria, and direct intervention in the management of that patient will take place to assure quality.
2. The quality of medical care can be assured in a more indirect fashion by conducting retrospective assessment of patterns of care, with the data derived from this inspection then forming a basis for continuing medical education programs designed to correct the deficiencies uncovered in the audit process.

Since it can be argued that quality assurance, through direct intervention in individual instances of care, can only be defended if the review system is better informed about all aspects of the patient's problem than is the physician being reviewed, and since it is untenable for a

PSRO to make such a claim of superior knowledge of each patient's case, one could extrapolate the PSRO mandate to a requirement, by PSROs, for continuing medical education, which would make the transference from quality assessment to quality assurance. If this assumption is correct, it follows that the PSRO must also evaluate the effectiveness of its education programs to justify the expenditure of public monies for this area of activity.

Common misconceptions could be held in peer review circles regarding the link between quality assessment and CME. The first of these is the fallacy that a quality audit automatically results in behavior change. The second is that the primary direction of formalized CME can be realistically guided by medical audit. There is some experience from which these conclusions are derived.

In 1972, the Utah Professional Review Organization (UPRO) began medical audit against process criteria, which had been specifically designed by specialty panels to be critical to ideal care. Criteria for establishing criticality were developed; and after the criteria were in rough draft form, staff concentrated on making the criteria more precise and rendering all criteria answerable with a yes-no response. A computerized data system was developed that produced compliance reports for each criterion for the entire system, for each hospital in comparison with other hospitals, and for the individual physicians. These reports were produced for each of over twenty diagnoses subject to audit.

Registered nurse coordinators, who were doing screening and data collection as part of the utilization review program, also collected the data for the quality audit. Inspection of these data quickly disclosed unmet criteria to serve as the basis for corrective education because of both the importance to patient outcome and the prevalence of noncompliance.

The printouts detailing physician performance were sent to each hospital staff and were reviewed by the specialty panels which set the criteria. Each specialty panel was instructed to review the compliance for each of the criteria and either find it acceptable, suggest education programs if compliance was not acceptable, or request a literature search if doubt existed. Furthermore, a representative of the audit committee for each of the participating hospitals was asked to discuss the findings of the medical audits at staff and department meetings and to report on the outcome of the discussion. The representative was also asked to submit suggestions for study improvements.

Some of the audit results were published in the *Bulletin* of the Utah State Medical Association. Others formed the subject of state specialty meetings. In an effort to make the education program more precise, seven criteria, the validity of which was thought to be unquestioned, were selected for intensive education; and efforts to catalyze hospital staff discussions around these specific criteria were redoubled. Despite these efforts, changes in physician behavior were negligible. Furthermore, vast amounts of data were collected without any subsequent useful application.

Why was this so? Upon analysis, process criteria elements appear to be placed into three categories by the target physicians when the results of audit are revealed:

1. Criteria, which although critical to ideal care, represent so obvious an action that audit is unnecessary. (Example: Did the physician take a history of chest pain in a patient with myocardial infarction?)
2. Criteria which are of questionable validity. (Example: Plasma renin determination in patients studied for hypertension.)
3. Criteria which appear to have little impact on patient outcome. (Example: Family history in patients with diabetes.)

The physician panels responsible for generating criteria received the compliance data and, in many cases, performed thoughtful and constructive critiques of the data. The next step, that of transferring the critiques into a general awareness of apparent deficits with subsequent change in professional performance was by and large a disappointment for our peer review program. Because of the above factors, the reports generated by peer review activity were either rejected or ignored as being irrelevant to patient outcome, or as having applied to an anonymous physician population which did not include the individual recipient of the data. The earlier efforts at behavior modification were handicapped by not being proximate or personal enough to create the desired impact. This experience also suggests an expected degree of skepticism by hospitals over the accuracy of the data collection methods, although reaudit has shown a concordance exceeding 95 percent.

As a result of these factors, the flow of CME opportunities from the quality assessment experience was much lighter than had been expected; therefore, the approach was changed from disease studies to medical audit two years ago. The audits now exclusively involve special projects selected because they possess a potential for continuing education, as well as representing areas where physician performance should be improved. Studies such as an audit of hospital complications, one of surgery for breast cysts , a study of indications for in-patient cystoscopy, and one on whole blood transfusion all provide data that can be used directly for education. When UPRO does conduct disease-oriented studies, they are based on "management objectives," which are more concise and have more relevance to patient outcome.

Thus, the PSRO quality assessment activity has been gradually, but substantially, altered, with the stimulus for change being the need for more applicability to CME. The program now seeks to make education more direct and proximate, utilizing the contact between reviewing and attending physician in a one-on-one relationship, supported by accepted criteria. Studies now center on issues that alter management of a particular case when criteria are not met. Efforts in this area must be cautious ones, and only be for specific studies, such as one being conducted for anemia. The reason for this is obvious: the quality of medical care would be impaired if diagnosis-oriented process audits were used in an intervention mode because the review system cannot hope to know as much about each individual patient as does the attending physician.

Most PSROs are identifying one particular committee to receive peer review data and construct appropriate education programs. The Utah State Medical Association (USMA) recognized the magnitude of this task early and formed a sister corporation of UPRO to perform this function. The Utah Academy of Continuing Medical Education (ACME) was organized and funded by USMA, with additional support from UPRO. The governing board of ACME contains representatives of USMA, UPRO, the Utah State Licensing Board, the University of Utah School of Medicine, and experts in educational research and data processing. It has its own staff. A primary objective is to construct CME programs to answer deficiencies revealed by UPRO audit.

While ACME is filling an ever-expanding continuing education role, much of the real education in PSRO activity will not lend itself to formalized or structured education techniques. It will have to be intuitive, reflecting the initiative of the hospital audit committees, and will be directed toward the poorest performing physicians.

This probably is not all bad. It is difficult to see how PSROs and hospital staff committees can compete effectively with the plethora of free education agents, conceived by educational research specialists, and backed by the resources of the advertising sponsor. The throw-away journal is probably the most effective medical education source in the country today, with audio-digest tapes a close second. There is reason to suggest that a PSRO should emphasize its capability to uncover and correct really poor care and collect data to identify the causes of problems in the system (i.e., why do patients fall out of bed?). PSROs should abandon, for now, efforts to develop postgraduate courses based on audit findings or to restructure medical school curricula. These latter goals realistically might not be achievable.

EDUCATION IN UTILIZATION REVIEW

Utilization review itself has substantial education potential, since physician actions governing patient admission and length of stay have often been intuitive or based on previous instruction that was also not validated by clinical research. The decision to admit a patient to the hospital for diagnostic investigation for hypertension, for initial regulation of diabetes, or for endocrinologic studies might have been governed by convenience to the patient or physician, or for personal economic factors rather than the need for acute hospital care. More efficient habits can be taught by the review system — most effectively through searching and tactful questioning by the reviewer, bolstered by peer-consensus criteria, and ultimately by the possibility of claim denial.

Length of stay, also, has often been determined by bias rather than solid clinical studies. Thus, the length of stay for myocardial infarction varies from fourteen days in some PSRO areas to twenty-eight days in others.

Finally, indications for elective surgery are sometimes fuzzy, often dictated by patient demands rather than solid consensus criteria and careful consideration of all practical options. "Cookbook medicine" is not the issue. Rather, a sense of conscience and consideration of all factors necessary for a practical allocation of the available health care dollar provide the milieu for effective education of provider and patient alike.

THE ROLE OF PSRO IN CONSUMER EDUCATION

PSROs have a significant, and largely unexploited, opportunity to educate patients. One area that requires greater effort is an attempt to teach patients about the potential value of peer review, both to curtail unnecessary medical cost, and to provide quality assurance.

Another obligation of PSRO is to encourage public education programs that provide a more informed and rational selection, by the patient, of level-of-care alternatives. This includes an honest explanation to the patient of the scope and intent of benefits offered by federally sponsored medical insurance programs. Our patients too often have gross misconceptions of what kinds of long-term care, for instance, are offered by their Medicare coverage.

EVALUATION OF CME PROGRAMS

When PSROs are responsible for launching CME programs, the evaluation of those programs is easily and logically carried out by reaudit. Indeed, unless reassessment shows behavior change, the entire system is indicted. Furthermore, the direction of change must benefit patients, either directly or indirectly. Unfortunately, most PSROs currently seem to be rushing to satisfy an urge to use some kind of criteria to measure someone's performance, without seriously considering what they are going to do with the data. Will it be usable? How? And to what ultimate purpose?

Part IV
Financial Aspects of CME

Chapter 12
Benefit-Cost Aspects of
Continuing Medical Education

Alan C. Monheit

The growing concern with the quality of care delivered by the U.S. health care system has prompted a number of responses from health specialists and professionals. Among the more important recommendations, policies incorporating continuing medical education have received much attention. Indeed, medical professionals seem so certain of the ameliorative effects of increased doses of continuing education that they have convinced a number of states and professional societies to adopt CME as a requirement for recertification or membership. As of this writing, for example, some fourteen state medical associations and six specialty societies are in the process of implementing CME participation as a condition for membership. In addition, the medical practice acts of nine states provide the state board of medical examiners with authority to require CME for reregistration of medical licensure. Furthermore, since all twenty-two specialty boards will require recertification in the near future, CME will likely serve as a prerequisite for such action.[1]

The resultant growth in CME participation is testimony to organized medicine's capacity to galvanize resources when a need is perceived. In the five-year period between 1969 and 1974, total physician registration in CME programs grew at an annual rate of 13.2 percent. The number of individual physicians in that total grew by 17.7 percent, and the number of courses actually presented by over 12 percent.[2] In 1970, for example, roughly one physician in three participated in CME programs; by 1974 this figure had nearly doubled.[3] Given this rapid response, however, it is a curious fact that little analytical effort has been directed to the issue of whether the *costs* (private and social) of such participation are justified by the *benefits* that are perceived to emanate from these programs. Although a thorough empirical evaluation is admittedly difficult and beyond the scope of this essay, it is my purpose to offer some insight into the factors that should enter such an analysis. In addition, I hope to raise some questions regarding the appropriateness of formal CME structures as a means of assuring physician quality. Since CME efforts can be viewed as an investment activity utilizing scarce resources, the calculus of benefit-cost analysis will provide a general framework for the investigation.

The plan of this chapter is as follows: a brief guide to the principles of benefit-cost analysis will be followed by a detailed discussion of the benefits and costs of CME programs. Some issues will then be explored regarding equity and efficiency in the administration of CME programs, followed by general conclusions.

BENEFIT-COST ANALYSIS: SOME GENERAL PRINCIPLES

The application of benefit-cost analysis[4] to an assessment of CME programs recognizes that such programs may be construed largely as *investment activities*. Such activities involve postponing the use of resources for current consumption purposes so a flow of future benefits (e.g., goods and services) can be received. Thus the calculus of benefit-cost analysis establishes a framework through which an evaluation can be made of the merits and costs of particular investment projects, along with a criterion for selection among alternative projects. Although benefit-cost analysis has been applied primarily by decision makers in the public sector, its principles are entirely consistent with those governing private investment decisions.

As its overriding principle, benefit-cost analysis asserts that in selecting a particular investment project, or level of investment within a project, a choice should be made that maximizes *net benefits* (the surplus of benefits over cost). The appropriate level of a given investment, therefore, should lie where the marginal benefits from the last unit of output produced equal the marginal costs of producing that level of activity. Given the scarcity of investment resources, investment priorities are established among a number of alternatives by enumerating benefit-cost ratios and selecting, *by order of magnitude*, those above unity. (Thus the projects selected are those with the largest benefit per dollar cost.) For consistent evaluations to be made, therefore, a guide for classifying benefits and costs must be established.

Although the goal of benefit-cost analysis is based upon a rather straightforward conceptualization, proper assessment of both benefits and costs requires great care and is often fraught with arbitrariness and disagreement over magnitudes. A correct accounting of benefits and costs must avoid elements that only reflect changes in income distribution (changes in resource control, prices, and transfer payments, for example) and thus concentrate on policy ramifications that alter productivity, avert costs, and cause resources to be harnessed for project construction and maintenance. In addition, imputations should be made for both "psychic" benefits and costs of projects, since these intangibles also affect individual welfare and must not be ignored. Finally, both benefits and costs must recognize effects on third parties, or "indirect" or external effects.

As the above discussion has indicated, therefore, the benefits of a project can take several forms. The most obvious element in this category consists of gains in productivity (real output) that would appear if the project were undertaken. A less obvious candidate for inclusion is *averted resource costs.* If the implementation of the project frees resources for use in the production of other goods and services, then such averted costs clearly should be included among the project benefits. Inclusion of psychic benefits recognizes improvements in welfare resulting from the project, although imputations of the value of such benefits are difficult to ascertain. An important point to note is that price changes that favor some individuals are not to be included as benefits, since *other* individuals will experience a decline in welfare. These changes, along with any transfer payments, are viewed as alterations in the distribution of income that ultimately balance out and do not change general welfare.

In a similar manner, the evaluation of costs should include the value of real resources used (hence productive opportunities sacrificed) in project development. These include direct costs for project construction and operation, as well as transaction costs involved in program administration. In addition, psychic costs should be included, since these reflect detriments to individual welfare. Finally, any costs borne by third parties that cause alterations in their behavior should be included, subject to the general guidelines developed above.

An important feature of the benefit-cost framework is the explicit recognition of the time structure of both benefits and costs. Since benefits and costs received or incurred in the future are worth "less" than similar dollar amounts currently received, each flow must be properly discounted to account for differences in their time paths.

Thus the benefit-cost comparisons actually made are between present discounted values. That is,

$$PDVB = \sum_{i=1}^{n} \frac{Bi}{(1+r)^i} \quad ; \quad PDVC = \sum_{i=1}^{n} \frac{Ci}{(1+r)^i} \quad .$$

In these expressions *PDVB*, *PDVC* are, respectively, present values of benefits and costs; *Bi* and *Ci* are benefits and costs in the ith period; and *r* is the rate of discount. Since there is considerable controversy among economists regarding the appropriate rate of discount, present values are estimated for a number of interest rate values. The notion of time structure of benefits and costs is particularly important since the selection among alternatives can depend vitally upon when these flows are expected to be received. For example, if one project has a large benefit package that is expected to be received far in the future, its present value could fall short of a project with a smaller flow of benefits received earlier. As I shall discuss below, the gain from investments in education among existing physicians could well depend on the distribution of the physicians' age and hence the length of time during which benefits are expected to flow.

With this brief survey of the general principles of benefit-cost analysis completed, the reader can now turn to an assessment of the specific benefits and costs emanating from CME programs. It is my contention that the costs of such a method of quality assurance are both large and real—but that the benefits might be somewhat more illusory.

BENEFITS OF CME PROGRAMS

Although CME activities can take a number of forms (self-assessment exams, traditional classroom lectures, independent study, and formal conferences, to note several modes), this discussion will pay most attention to formal programs of instruction. In general, such CME activities can be classified as either review-oriented or designed to impart knowledge of new techniques of diagnosis or treatment. Included in the former might be programs somewhat more punitive in nature, directed at physicians who have been judged by their peers to fall below minimal standards of sound medical practice. In general, therefore, the benefits emanating from CME programs will depend on the nature of each type of program. This discussion will therefore outline the *private* and *social* benefits of each. An analysis of the costs will follow.

Benefits from Review-Oriented CME Programs

For the most part, benefits emanating from this class of programs can be viewed as taking the form of *averted resource costs*. Private benefits or returns from investment by an individual practitioner will, therefore, first consist of losses avoided from declines in productivity.* That is, such activities might aid the physician in repairing any depreciation that his human capital might have experienced in various areas of his practice. This could range from review of diagnostic procedures to techniques for avoiding "managerial slack" in the organization of one's medical practice. To the extent that such programs are able to curtail and reverse declines in productivity, the physician-student will avoid losses to his medical practice. (It is important to note that such private returns accrue to society in the physician's role as a member of society. By social returns and costs we will refer to those elements borne by remaining or nonphysician components.) In addition, to the degree that such review-oriented CME activities prevent physicians from making improper diagnoses and therefore extending improper medical care, "transactions" costs associated with malpractice contingencies will be averted. These include costs of litigation (legal fees, possible court costs, and penalties), associated time costs (preparation for and participation in legal action) and obvious psychic costs. The level of such costs would lie far above those reflected in current malpractice premiums paid by physicians.

A final element that should be recognized as a valid part of private returns consists of any psychic returns from participation in CME activities. These returns are a composite of both investment and "consumption" aspects implicit in such participation: for example, any enhancement of professional stature (such as the Physician's Recogni-

---

*Note that if CME programs are entirely voluntary, participation by an individual physician is akin to an investment decision or a private benefit-cost calculation (with both private and social returns and costs). The movement toward mandatory CME reflects society's judgment that such private investments have the potential of generating a sufficiently large volume of social returns, but that the current level of private returns fails to stimulate an optimal level of investment. This has implications for allocating the financial burden of such programs. Note also that this emphasis does not preclude consideration of consumption aspects of CME activities.

tion Award discussed in Chapter 1) or enjoyment of CME sessions (e.g., contacts made or location of conference). One would therefore expect the physician-investor to consider such returns in his private benefit-cost evaluation.

The returns to *society* (i.e., consumers of medical services) emanating from such review-oriented CME activities consist of several distinct components. As Charles Phelps has suggested elsewhere,[5] a conceptually important benefit derived from attempts to assure quality entails the avoidance of potential resource losses due to *misinformation* conveyed by physicians. Such misinformation can result in misallocations of such scarce resources as physician and patient time, as well as complementary medical inputs. To the extent that such misinformation (and hence misallocations) are avoided, society captures productivity gains from a "correct" (i.e., efficient) utilization of resources. Part of this gain encompasses the time structure of real output. That is, by correctly diagnosing and treating those with illnesses, society captures productive contributions that might otherwise be postponed to future periods. (Such postponement could result from two interrelated causes: misdiagnosis and/or mistreatment will defer correct diagnosis and treatment to future periods, thereby contributing to a further deterioration of the individual's health status. As a result, real productive contributions by these individuals will be deferred.) To the extent that physician time is more efficiently utilized, more patients can be seen/treated with productivity gains accruing both to society and to the physician.

Finally, a source of psychic returns is also present in these societal benefits. Some returns are derived from society's desire to have an "inventory" of practitioners of relatively constant quality. That is, since recipients of medical care are most likely to be "risk averse" with regard to sources from which they purchase care,* any reduction in risk associated with a reduction in the variance of quality will enhance utility.

The above, then, comprises a set of benefits believed to be associated with review-oriented CME programs. Rather than comment at this point on the impact such benefits are likely to have, that discussion will be deferred until a similar enumeration of the benefits associated with a second class of CME activities is presented.

---

*A risk averse individual, if confronted with a choice between a payoff obtained with *certainty* and one with the same expected value obtained through a "gamble," would select the former.

Benefits of CME Programs Designed to Introduce
Physicians to Advances in Diagnosis and Treatment

CME programs included in this category might be viewed as activities whose goal is to upgrade physician quality beyond minimal or current levels of acceptability. As such, the programs have a distinct set of private and social benefits. Private benefits accruing to the practitioner consist largely of opportunities for increased productivity (and hence pecuniary gain) derived from the potential application of such new techniques. To the extent that more effective treatment of existing patients can be enhanced, such activities enable the physician to broaden his scope of practice, with new patients seeking such treatment.* In addition to such productivity-enhancing private benefits, psychic returns such as those recognized above will also enter the calculus of private returns. Included in such returns could be the physician's own satisfaction that his practice exemplifies the current mode of "quality" medical care.

Societal benefits generated by this class of CME activities are governed by the degree to which the infusion of such new technology permits the capture of otherwise lost productivity. Such gains could be obtained through more effective treatment of the chronically ill, from postponing (or leveling out the rate of) depreciation of human capital, or from reducing diagnosis and/or treatment time. An additional component for consideration among these social benefits are psychic returns. These returns are implicit in society's desire to achieve "Cadillac" level medical care by maintaining an "inventory" of up-to-date practitioners. The emergency and uncertain nature of medical care, in which care less than that of the highest quality is often regarded as equivalent to no care, is also a source for this type of benefit.

Before attempting to assess the impact of such benefits, it should be noted that implicit in attempts to implement CME programs are returns that accrue to organized medicine.[6] As such, their nature deserves a brief comment. The development of formal CME structures, for example, is one way of establishing and maintaining lines of communication and discipline between organized medicine and the existing population of practicing physicians. More important (and pro-

---

*While pecuniary gains from possible referrals could enter the physician's private benefit calculations, it should be noted that referrals *per se* constitute a form of income redistribution that "washes out" when one considers social benefits. If one physician is gaining referrals, then other physicians, it stands to reason, are losing referrals. Overall, the net effects of such a redistribution of referrals could approach zero.

vocative), the establishment of such activities serves to enable organized medicine to defer the costs of more rigorous regulatory mechanisms, such as periodic reexamination requirements, to future generations of physicians. Both these elements enable organized medicine to exercise more direct control over attempts to regulate medical practice. Clearly, attempts to legitimatize CME via mandatory provisions could be interpreted as one manifestation of this desire to retain control.

The Impact of CME Benefits: A Caveat

While the benefits enumerated above might appear to have the potential for a large contribution to social welfare, I believe that great care must be exercised in appraising their magnitude. In particular, it is my belief that these benefits might be somewhat illusory, especially when the costs of establishing formal CME structures are considered.

Since medical care is generally characterized by uncertainty, it is not at all clear that the benefits from CME will flow with any degree of consistency. That is, the flow of such benefits is governed by probability distributions. Underlying such distributions is the frequency with which CME applications will occur. An implication of viewing the benefit flow in this manner is that there is no guarantee that the expected value of benefits in each period will be of a magnitude comparable with the costs (which are required to flow each period). In particular, there could be a considerable disparity between the information conveyed in CME programs and the opportunities physicians have to apply such information. This will be true in both review-oriented CME activities as well as those designed to impart new knowledge. As regards the former, there will be substantial differences in the flow of benefits if the majority of physicians choose this form of participation (as they might to meet a mandatory nuisance provision), or if those physicians judged as practicing below standard quality medicine (and most likely to benefit from such programs) are required to attend. With respect to the latter type of program, the patient population served by the physician might offer scant opportunity to utilize the new medical technology he has acquired. Whether this will generate frustration and attempts to "over-doctor" (i.e., infuse the new technology) is an issue that must be considered. Finally, and perhaps most important, it is not at all evident that CME participation *per se* will guarantee quality: that attendance (whether voluntary or mandatory) without some burden of proof regarding knowledge acquisition will be translated into improved quality in the provision of care. In light of the above, I would urge research efforts to be directed toward more specific and empirical evaluations of the benefits forthcoming from CME activities.[7] Such research efforts should also be extended to establish quantifiable indices of health status. Since physician participation in CME is ostensibly designed to improve the quality (and hence efficacy) of care, the development of such indices would provide a complementary measure with which to assess the benefits from CME participation.

Given these caveats, this author is not at all confident that benefits are commensurate with efforts to induce formal CME structures. The costs, however, are certain to be incurred—and their magnitude is likely to be substantial. It is to a discussion of these costs that this chapter now turns.

COSTS OF CME

Since the costs associated with either type of CME program are similar, this discussion will point out some of the direct costs to practitioners and the social (external) costs involved in CME implementation.

Direct Costs to Medical Practitioners

Involved in any educational effort are certain costs borne directly by participants. An obvious component of such costs are any fees, tuition, book expenses, or other related entry costs (e.g., transportation costs). In general, such costs are usually minor when compared with a less obvious component: the opportunity or "time" costs of earnings that are forgone from participation in CME activities. These costs will be substantial and are certain to be incurred during each period of CME participation.[8] Note that it is not valid to argue that such time could be drawn from leisure, rendering the time costless. The choice of an hour of leisure also involves a cost: the wage one forgoes by not working. As shall be discussed below, it is not unreasonable to assume that the imposition of a mandatory CME requirement would induce physicians to allocate time away from work, toward leisure and CME participation.

Social Costs of CME

The social costs of continuing medical education consist of costs borne by consumers of health services along with other members of society. The estimation of such costs does not lend itself as readily as an approximation of the direct time costs, therefore the following discussion will be primarily conceptual.

Among those social costs that should be recognized are those arising directly from physician participation in CME. As noted above, these could include added resource costs of treatment when more expensive, CME-inspired modes of care (which are either unnecessary or do not improve health outcomes) are used. Once again, this refers to the "technological imperative" inherent in medical care and the potential hazard of "over-doctoring" that could result from CME participation. In addition, physician time spent in formal CME activities involves deferred treatment of patients and hence a postponement of real output (produced by patients) to future periods. Included among the costs of deferred treatment are the obvious psychic costs borne by patients and their families.

In addition to the costs cited above, CME participation could inadvertently foster a tendency that the medical profession and society at large are trying to avoid: the loss of interest in general medical practice and concentration in areas of "superspecialization."[9] Such a tendency could also result in costs borne by consumers of health care: psychic costs reflecting dissatisfaction with available care, as well as time costs involved as consumers search or acquire information regarding the physician most appropriate for their particular ailments. In an era in which there seems to be a considerable maldistribution of physicians by specialty,[10] such costs would be far from negligible.

Other costs that should be recognized as borne by society at large fall under the general heading of "transactions" costs. These include the use of resources to administer and enforce (especially with respect to mandatory CME) CME activities; costs of identifying "incompetent" physicians (if in fact review-oriented CME programs are to be more "punitive" in nature); and costs of evaluating the efficacy of CME structures (such costs are almost always incurred when new programs are implemented). In addition, if tuition and fees are not sufficient to cover program costs, it is quite likely (and equitable) that public funding will be utilized. Hence portions of other public projects could be sacrificed. Finally, since CME programs will require the use of physician-instructors, society will forgo any difference between their productivity in medical practice and their productivity as instructors.

There is one less obvious social cost inherent in any attempt to compel physician participation in continuing education. To the extent that such programs are mandatory, a large social cost could be encountered if physicians in the upper end of the age distribution decide not to make the required investment. Note that the size of this group is not unsubstantial: in 1973, for example, over 25 percent of physicians were of age 55 or above.[11] It is a well-known aspect of the theory of human capital that the incentive to invest declines with age.[12] Hence, it is not unreasonable to suspect that some physicians in this group will evaluate the returns from such additional investments as "too low" (this will depend upon the group's current and expected future participation in medical practice). Given such circumstances, will society choose to bar these practitioners from medical practice? If so, the social costs from the loss of such accumulated knowledge and experience may be substantial. (An implication of this analysis, therefore, is that CME programs should have some flexibility with regard to physician characteristics.)

To conclude this discussion, it must be reemphasized that such costs can be expected to be incurred in each period with a greater degree of certainty than the expected flow of benefits. Furthermore, given attempts to mandate the time required for CME participation, one suspects that such costs will also be substantial. With these factors in mind, I would seriously question any assertion that the benefit-cost ratio would exceed unity. Finally, there are difficulties inherent in the actual measurement of certain benefit-cost components. They do exist, but they probably do not constitute a valid basis for criticism. Rather, the benefit-cost approach enables a number of relevant and viable policy considerations to be raised that might otherwise easily go undetected.

EQUITY AND EFFICIENCY IN CME

The ultimate use of benefit-cost analysis is to provide a framework for assessing the relative merits of competing investment projects. Often, however, the process of benefit-cost analysis raises issues regarding both the equity and efficiency with which resources will be used to implement desired projects. Equity is the way in which resource use can affect the distribution of income or welfare; efficiency is the manner in which resources are applied: will they yield a maximum level of output? Four considerations need to be explored: the burden of the costs of financing CME, the effect of mandatory CME on physician time allocation and hence the flow of services, the question of whether all age groups should have uniform requirements, and the relationship between desired quality of care and periodic continuing education.

Financing CME Programs

The current tendency to legislate or prescribe hour requirements for CME programs suggests that voluntary efforts by physicians fall below the level desired by society. In particular, this reveals a disparity between private and social benefits of CME activities, validating assertions presented above. Since optimality in the provision of an activity is attained when the marginal benefits (both private and social) from the last unit of said activity equal the marginal costs (again both private and social), it is not clear that physicians as a group should bear the costs of financing CME activities. This is illustrated in Figure 12-1, which presents a simple model of the demand and supply for continuing education. The vertical axis represents dollar values of marginal benefits and costs, and the horizontal axis represents the quantity of CME (measured either in hours or number of courses). Demand schedule D_p represents the private demand for continuing education by physicians as a group: that is, each point on the schedule

Figure 12-1

SIMPLE MODEL OF CME DEMAND AND SUPPLY

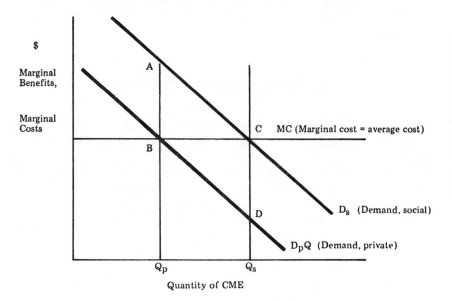

Quantity of CME

reflects the marginal benefit forthcoming to physicians from the last unit of CME purchased. Demand schedule D_S adds social benefits to private benefits and therefore reflects the *full* social benefits from additional CME (any point on D_S approximates the marginal social benefit from additional units of CME). Schedule MC reflects the marginal costs of producing additional units of CME. For simplicity, this cost is assumed to be constant and to reflect the incremental resource costs involved in providing an additional unit of CME (assumed to be reflected in tuition and fees).

Optimality is achieved for physicians (as a group) at point B and output Q_p, where the marginal private benefits and costs are equal. However, social optimality is achieved at point C and output Q_S, where the full marginal benefits (private and social) equal marginal costs. If society mandates level Q_S but requires physicians to bear the additional costs, physicians will suffer a loss in welfare while the remaining members of society will gain. This can be shown as follows: by moving from Q_p to Q_S, physicians achieve a gain in total utility of area BDQ_SQ_p; however, they also incur an extra cost of area BCQ_SQ_p.* Note that since area BCQ_SQ_p (added costs) exceeds area BDQ_SQ_p (added benefits), physicians experience a welfare loss of area BCD. The rest of society, however, receives an increment in welfare by moving from point A to point C (a gain in total utility of area $ACDB$).** As a result of this compulsion, welfare is redistributed with physicians the net losers and the rest of society net gainers.

There is, however, a way to redress this apparent inequity. From Figure 12-1 it is evident that the gainers can, in fact, compensate the losers for their decline in welfare. Note that the area of welfare gain $ACDB$ exceeds the area of welfare loss BCD. An improvement in social welfare would therefore require that the gainers be able to compensate the losers so no one is left worse off by the resource reallocation.*** Given the geometry of the gains and losses, it is evident that

---

*The area under a demand curve reflects the total utility or satisfaction associated with the interval of purchases. Since marginal cost is assumed to be constant, it equals average cost. Therefore, the change in total cost equals the product of the constant average cost and the change in quantity.

**Parallelogram $ACDB$ constitutes the gain in utility to the rest of society by increasing the level of CME from Q_p to Q_S. This is derived by noting that the vertical distance between D_S and D_p reflects marginal social (nonphysician) benefits, and that the cost component, BCD, is being borne by physicians.

***This is an application of the "compensation principle" derived from the economist's notion of Pareto Optimality. Pareto Optimality argues that a gain in social welfare will be achieved (from an alteration in resource allocation) if at least one party is made better off with no one being made worse off.

such a compensation can be made, with society gaining welfare equivalent to area *ACB*. In particular, this implies that the rest of society should bear the costs of financing any additional CME it deems necessary (in excess of the level determined optimal by private decision makers). Such cost sharing is in the interest of equity and, hence, social welfare. (To the extent that the federal government provides tax incentives for CME, some cost sharing does exist.)

CME and Physician Time Allocation

If physicians were free to choose the amount of time to allocate to CME activities, one would expect them to do so in a manner consistent with utility maximization. That is, the achievement of such a private optimum would reflect an equality, at the margin, between utility per dollar expenditure on all uses of time: work, leisure, and continuing education time. The imposition of mandatory CME time requirements would, however, distort this private optimum and lead physicians to reallocate their time decisions in a manner consistent with the requirement. The effect of such a reallocation could have serious consequences for physician working time and hence for the production of

The relationship between mandatory CME and the physician's decision to allocate time to hours of work can be explored by drawing from the economist's theory of labor supply. This theory has components that can be used to explain time allocation in both a one-period and life cycle framework. Consider the physician's behavior in a one-period (static) framework. Consistent with real world behavior, one might expect the physician to allocate the largest proportion of his time to work, with the remainder (assuming free choice) divided between leisure and CME time. Given both the quantity and quality (intensity) of physician work time, one might expect the marginal utility (i.e., added satisfaction) from the last hour of work to fall below the utility of the last hour allocated to leisure or CME.* If a mandatory CME time

---

*Here the author assumes diminishing marginal utility or satisfaction: as more time is allocated to a particular activity, the addition to satisfaction, or marginal utility, declines. The conclusions derived from this application of labor supply theory can all be rigorously demonstrated. In the above one-period application, CME time provides utility to the physician, where such utility can reflect productive and psychic rewards. Note that this is not inconsistent with viewing CME as an investment activity, for these aspects will be captured in a life cycle labor supply model. By treating CME time as a component of utility, the one-period model can be used, and plausible results can be obtained consistent with the former investment emphasis.

requirement were imposed, therefore, we would expect that the physician would draw hours to meet the requirement from the source whose marginal utility of time was low: *work time.* In doing so, his loss in total utility (satisfaction) would be minimized. Thus, it is not unreasonable to expect working time to decline in light of a mandatory CME time requirement.* In a life cycle context, furthermore, CME participation could also lead to a postponement of some portion of working time to future periods. If such current investment leads to future wage increases, life cycle labor supply theory unambiguously predicts a reallocation of lifetime hours of work to future periods.[13]

The main point of this digression, therefore, is to recognize that mandating or encouraging CME activities could have an impact regarding *when* medical care will be received. Thus an important aspect for policy makers to consider is that CME activity could well influence the distribution of care between the present and future. As a result, some evaluation of social preferences regarding the timing of such care is required.

CME and Physician Characteristics:
The Issue of Physician Age

An important component of social costs associated with CME is the effect such programs can have on those physicians in the upper tail of the age distribution (especially when confronted by mandatory CME). A closely related issue entails decisions by society involving the use of resources to improve quality in younger and older workers.[14] In particular, an effort by society to use resources for educational efforts to improve quality also involves consideration as to which group is most "profitable" in deciding where to concentrate the efforts. Since the flow of quality from investments made in younger workers will exceed the flow emanating from older workers (assuming costs of investments and quality per period to be the same), there will be a "social loss" for each dollar invested in an older worker. This is not to say that there should be no resources allocated to assure quality in older workers; rather, society should be aware that these costs exist when such allocations are made. The issue of age points to the fact that different physician groups should be treated with respect to their specific needs, while acknowledging the benefits and costs associated with resource

---

*Leisure time can also *increase* under certain assumptions. A demonstration of this point is available from the author upon request.

allocation toward each group. It might be that a uniform program is one for which the social costs are the largest.

The Relationship Between Desired Quality, Actual Quality, and Periodic Continuing Education

An important issue regarding the optimal implementation of CME programs entails the frequency with which physicians should be required to participate. Since such activities involve considerable costs (especially time costs), attempts should be made to economize on the frequency of physician participation. This frequency will depend on the relationship between the path of physician quality (the actual quality of a physician at any given point in time) and the level of quality desired by society. In general, the greater the level of desired quality, the more frequently physicians will be required to participate in CME activities and, therefore, the larger the costs.

Consider the time paths displayed in Figure 12-2. $Q(t)$ represents the time path of physician quality and is hypothesized to rise throughout the period of formal medical school training and peak (point B) several years beyond internship or residency. With no CME (i.e., increments to investment in human capital), one might expect quality to decline as, for example, bad practice habits develop or the physician fails to recognize or include new medical technology.* $S(t)$ represents the path of quality desired by society and is assumed to represent the minimum socially acceptable level of quality. Its path is assumed to rise over-time, as new technology is infused into health care delivery. Note that point A can be viewed as representing graduation from medical school: the point at which the physician first meets society's minimal quality standards.

Consider now point C, at which the intersection between actual and desired quality is achieved. Beyond this point actual quality falls below desired quality. Therefore, society would judge the physician as falling below minimal standards. Hence, one could expect CME to be pre-

---

*This description of the path of physician quality is admittedly extreme. For example, I assume that depreciation of quality outweighs any gains which might be made via experience in the physician's practice (portion of the schedule beyond B). However, one could postulate a model in which the rate of growth of quality declines over time (i.e., quality increases at a decreasing rate beyond some point) and in which the rate of growth in desired quality overtakes actual quality. The conclusions here would remain unchanged.

Figure 12-2

RELATIONSHIP BETWEEN PHYSICIAN QUALITY AND TIME

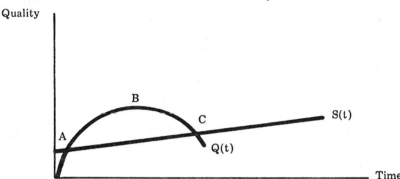

Figure 12-3

THE RELATIONSHIP BETWEEN PHYSICIAN QUALITY
AND TIME AFFECTED BY CME

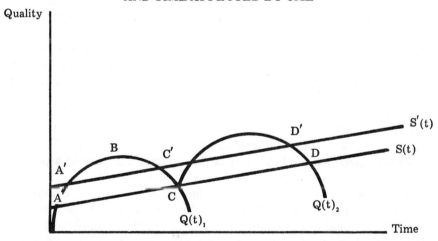

scribed as one way of redressing the deficiency.* Presumably, such an additional investment would generate another quality path resembling *Q(t)*. This is illustrated in Figure 12-3 by *Q(t)₂*. At a point such as *D* in Figure 12-3, additional investments would similarly be needed.

---

*The above model borrows from capital replacement theory, which describes the optimal point in time to replace capital whose productivity is depreciating. *C* also represents a point in time at which the present value of the surplus of actual quality over minimally acceptable quality is maximized.

The point of this digression is to note that if society's perceptions regarding the minimal level of quality were greater throughout time [i.e., $S'(t)$ in figure 12-3], more investments to ensure quality would be required throughout a physician's lifetime. Thus in Figure 12-3, examining now $S'(t)$, the length of medical school would increase, (A' exceeds A); and with C' occurring before C and D' before D (all points at which reinvestment would take place), more investment efforts would be required over a physician's life cycle. Correspondingly larger private and social costs would be incurred. As a result, society's desired level of quality will directly influence the magnitude of the forthcoming costs. Hence, such desired quality must be kept within reasonable limits.

CONCLUSION

The purpose of this chapter has been to raise conceptual issues regarding the benefits and costs involved in using continuing medical education as a means of assuring physician quality. From the issues discussed, it is this author's contention that the costs of such efforts (uniformly applied to all physicians) might easily outweigh the benefits. Such costs as have been identified are more likely to occur with a greater degree of certainty than the corresponding benefits. Until research efforts provide quantitative evidence concerning the relationship between benefits and costs, there should be far less emphasis on mandating CME requirements. Rather, if CME is to be used as a quality assurance mechanism, there should be greater attention given to ensuring that knowledge which may be transformed into improved practice quality is, in fact, acquired. The use of a periodic reexamination requirement, with correspondingly less emphasis on the *manner* in which the knowledge is acquired to demonstrate satisfactory performance, is one viable alternative.* Such a requirement would enable physicians to select the mode of continuing education most efficient for their own needs (i.e., formal or informal modes of instruction), thereby allowing both flexibility and potential cost savings to be achieved. In addition, such exams could be structured to

---

*It is a curious fact that while organized medicine relies heavily upon such mechanisms to ensure quality at the point of entry to medical practice (both for general and specialty practice), little use of these devices is made at points thereafter in the physician's career.

discover specific physician deficiencies (e.g., on the order of assessment exams) or be geared toward specific physician groups with particular characteristics. Finally, the payoff to such an activity, compared with traditional CME, might be enhanced, since at a minimum, some demonstration will be provided that the knowledge needed for strong correlation with quality of care has been acquired. Passing an exam does not guarantee that quality medical care will be delivered, but failure to pass an exam structured to detect deficiencies in such knowledge would strongly suggest that quality care has not been forthcoming.

NOTES

1. *Continuing Medical Education Fact Sheet* (American Medical Association, February 10, 1976).

2. Average Annual rates of growth computed from data in "Medical Education in the United States," *Journal of the American Medical Association* Supplement, various years.

3. *Ibid.* for participating physicians. Total physicians from *Reference Data on the Profile of Medical Practice* (Chicago: American Medical Association, 1971, 1974).

4. For a general survey of principles and issues in benefit-cost analysis, see E.J. Mishan, *Cost-Benefit Analysis*, (New York: Prager, 1974). For a survey of applications of benefit-cost analysis in health care, see Herbert Klarman, "Applications of Cost-Benefit Analysis to the Health Services and the Special Case of Technological Innovation," *International Journal of Health Services* 4, (1974): 325-352.

5. Charles Phelps, "Benefit-Cost Analysis of Quality Assurance Programs," in R.H. Egdahl and P.M. Gertman, eds., *Quality Assurance in Health Care* (Germantown, Md.: Aspen Systems Corp., 1976), p. 289.

6. I wish to thank Paul Gertman and Cynthia Taft for suggesting these possibilities.

7. For an example of such a research effort, see John W. Williamson, Marshall Alexander, and George E. Miller, "Continuing Education and Patient Care Research," *Journal of the American Medical Association* 201, (September 18, 1967): 118-122.

8. Using estimates obtained from AMA data, the hourly wage of a physician may range between $14.80 to over $23.00, depending upon specialty (hourly wages are constructed by dividing median yearly earnings by total hours worked during the year, where the latter figure is the product of average hours and average weeks worked per year). Source of data: *Reference Data on the Profile of Medical Practice* (AMA, 1971, 1974). It is obviously risky to offer predictions regarding the overall time costs involved, but if each active physician were required to attend between 30 to 50 hours of CME a year (as some mandatory legislation stipulates), such costs in the aggregate could range from $200 to $330 million.

9. On the relationship between "superspecialization" and access to quality medical care, see Robert A. Chase, M.D., "Proliferation of Certification in Medical Specialties: Productive or Counterproductive," *New England Journal of Medicine* 294, no. 9 (February 26, 1967): 497-499.

10. On this point see, for example, Frank Sloan, "Lifetime Earnings and Physicians' Choice of Specialty," *Industrial and Labor Relations Review* 24, (October 1970): 47-56.

11. *Profile of Medical Practice* (Chicago: American Medical Association, 1974), Table 26.

12. See the discussion in Gary S. Becker, *Human Capital,* 2nd ed. (New York: National Bureau of Economic Research, 1975), pp. 63-65. As age increases, the number of remaining periods to collect returns from additional investments declines, and the costs (income forgone) of such investment rise.

13. See Gary S. Becker and Gilert R. Ghez, *The Allocation of Time and Goods Over the Life Cycle* (New York: National Bureau of Economic Research, 1975), especially Chapter I. In essence the theory argues that, if the price of time (wage rate) is expected to rise in the future, less use of such time will be made for nonworking endeavors, and larger amounts of time will be allocated to work. Note that if the required time for CME is an uncertain element in life cycle decision making, an income effect (assumed not relevant with perfect certainty) may cause hours of work to *decline* over time (if the income effect exceeds the substitution effect).

14. For a comprehensive statement of the issues involved, see

Vladimir Stoikov, "Recurrent Education: Some Neglected Economic Issues," *International Labor Review* 108, (August-September 1973): 187-208.

Chapter 13
The Internal Revenue Code
and
Continuing Medical Education

Gregory T. Halbert

Although the continuing medical education requirements of the several states and specialty boards differ, they all have one thing in common — money. Doctors will have to spend it to take the CME courses necessary to retain their licenses to practice, or their specialty certification. This burden can, however, be mitigated under current federal income tax law, which allows a deduction for the ordinary and necessary expenses of doing business. As now written, the law includes most CME expenses in this category.

TAX LAW

Policy

The Internal Revenue Code (IRC) is associated in most minds with taxes to raise the revenue to finance government operations, and that is partially correct. However, tax law is also a policy tool that can be, and has been, used to direct taxpayer conduct toward national policy objectives by either encouraging or discouraging expenditures. This is accomplished through the allowance of deductions from gross income to determine taxable income, credits against the tax that is due, and preferential tax rates for certain types of income.

The policy of the federal government to encourage private ownership of homes is reflected by the IRC sections that allow a deduction for interest paid on mortgages,[1] and property taxes.[2] In 1975 Congress added section 44 to the IRC in an effort to bring the country out of the recession by stimulating the construction and purchase of new homes. It provided for a credit of "an amount equal to 5 percent of the purchase price of a new principal residence purchased or constructed by the taxpayer."[3] Another example of the use of tax laws to encourage national objectives is the political contribution provision. A credit of one-half of the contribution up to a maximum of $25 credit ($50 credit for a joint return) is allowed.[4] Preferred treatment of capital gains and losses is yet another example,[5] the policy here to stimulate capital investment in business and industry.

This dual purpose of the IRC must be kept in mind by policy makers, for adjustments to the IRC can be a potent tool to attain policy objectives totally unrelated to the revenue system. Changes in the deductibility of CME expenses can have a great impact on individual spending for CME, and hence on the mandatory nature of the program itself. For example, in tax year 1975, a married taxpayer filing a joint return reached the 50 percent marginal tax rate with a taxable income between $44,000 and $52,000. If we assume a taxable income of $45,000 and an expenditure of $1,000 for CME, there would be no marginal tax if the expense were deductible. If it were not deductible, there would be a marginal tax of $500 for a total CME cost of $1,500. The policy conclusion is obvious. If CME expenses were no longer deductible at all, or to the same extent as they now are, would mandatory CME remain a viable policy alternative to the national goal of improving the quality of medical care? The converse would be true if the deductibility of these expenses were liberalized. To aid CME policy makers to decide whether to utilize the potential of the IRC, this chapter will set out the law as it now is and also offer two proposals for change.

Business Expenses Deduction

It has long been part of the federal policy to provide an income tax incentive to taxpayers regarding the production of their income. This is not mandated by the Constitution, but it does make sense: if income is to be taxed, there will be more income subject to the tax if the government encourages more production. The remarks of Senator John Williams during a congressional debate on adoption of the first business expense deduction provision in 1913 explains this policy rationale:

> The object of this bill is to tax a man's net income; that is to say, what he has at the end of the year after deducting from his receipts his expenditures or losses.[6]

Section 162 of the IRC, which embodies this policy, states in pertinent part:

(a) IN GENERAL.— There shall be allowed as a deduction all the ordinary and necessary expenses paid or incurred during the taxable year in carrying on any trade or business, including—

(2) traveling expenses (including amounts expended for meals and lodging other than amounts which are lavish or extravagant under the circumstances) while away from home in the pursuit of a trade or business;

A change was made to this section in 1962 in response to abuses in the deduction of personal living expenses under the guise of business expenses. Prior to the amendment the phrase in parentheses read, "(including the entire amount expended for meals and lodging)." This change was necessitated because, as President John F. Kennedy said:

Too many firms and individuals have devised means of deducting too many personal living expenses as business expenses, thereby charging a large part of their cost to the Federal Government....

....Even though in some instances entertainment and related expenses have an association with the needs of business, they nevertheless confer substantial tax-free personal benefits to the recipients....[7]

The President had in mind section 262, which provides that:

Except as otherwise expressly provided in this chapter, no deduction shall be allowed for personal, living or family expenses.

CME EXPENSES

In the analysis of the deductibility of CME expenses there are five subareas that must be examined in detail: direct education expenses, travel, room and board, spouse's travel, and foreign travel.

Education

The law did not always recognize CME expenditures as an ordinary and necessary business expense qualifying for deduction. The Internal Revenue Service (IRS) issued an Income Tax Ruling in 1922 that:

> Expenses incurred by doctors in taking post-graduate
> courses are deemed to be in the nature of personal expenses
> and not deductible.[8]

However, the law has changed. IRS regulation § 1.162-5 now governs
the deduction of education expenses. A deduction is specifically allowed for, "refresher courses, courses dealing with current developments. . . ."[9] This will cover courses taken to satisfy requirements set
by speciality boards. Another section of the regulation allows a deduction for courses taken to meet the express requirements of law or
regulations imposed as a condition of continued employment or practice.[10]

The discretion that doctors have under this regulation in choosing
the courses they will take is illustrated by *Hill v. Commissioner of Internal Revenue.*[11] Mrs. Hill, a high school teacher in rural Virginia, was
required to either read five education texts from an approved list or attend summer school to keep her teaching certificate. She chose the
latter, and attended Columbia University. The commissioner denied
her deduction for the school expenses, saying that she had the burden
of proving that most other teachers in Virginia chose the summer
school alternative to satisfy the state requirement. The court chided
the commissioner for his attenuated argument and observed paren-
thetically that one of the courses she took, abnormal psychology, was
particularly well suited for a high school teacher. As long as the state
offered an alternative to the continued education requirement,
teachers were entitled to choose the one they preferred.

> If the particular course adopted by the taxpayer is a response
> that a reasonable person would normally and naturally make
> under the specific circumstances, that would suffice.[12]

The determination of what is an "ordinary" expense measures the
transaction out of which the expense arose against the business or profession of the taxpayer in which it occurred. As with all legal questions, the facts are all important. If Mrs. Hill instead had attended the
University of Hawaii and stayed on Waikiki Beach for a month after
the course ended, there would likely have been a different result.
However, it appears to be well-established law at this point that the
direct expense for mandatory CME is deductible under section 162.

Travel

Where it is necessary to travel to another city in the United States to attend a CME course, the expense associated with the travel is fully deductible if attendance at the CME course is the sole purpose of the trip. The same is true if the travel itself is taken as CME. However, complications arise when business is combined with personal pursuits that are unrelated to the taxpayer's business or profession. In the case of travel as a form of CME the entire travel expenditures will be deductible only if the "major portion of the activities during such period is of a nature which directly maintains or improves skills" required for the person's profession.[13]

Whether a particular trip is primarily for business purposes or primarily personal in nature, depends on all the facts and circumstances of each case. An important fact in this determination is the proportion of time spent on personal activity. Although there is no precise mathematical rule as to percent of time, given the fact that doctors (and lawyers) are reportedly the most frequently audited taxpayers, more than a 55 to 45 percent breakdown would probably be required for deductibility. The same basic rule applies to travel to another city to take a CME course. The major portion of the activities while in the visiting city must be related to CME if any of the travel expense is deductible.

Room and Board

The rule for deductibility of room and board is more lenient than that for travel expenses. Even if a trip is primarily for personal purposes, the room and board expenses for those days spent on CME is deductible, so long as the amounts are not "lavish or extravagant under the circumstances." The latitude that is permitted here is a recognition not only that living expenses in Boston are higher than they are in Dallas, for example, but that presidents will naturally prefer to stay in the presidential suite. However, if a taxpayer who is not a president stays in the presidential suite of his favorite hotel, he can expect to be audited.

Spouse's Expenses

Having thus covered the more straightforward situations, we can now proceed to the situation where the IRS regulation writers excel—

the spouses. The deductibility of a spouse's travel expenses (here meant to include both transportation and room and board) is governed by regulation §1.162-2(c):

> Where a taxpayer's wife (sic) accompanies him on a business trip, expenses attributable to her travel are not deductible unless it can be adequately shown that the wife's presence on the trip has a bona fide business purpose. The wife's performance of some incidental service does not cause her expenses to qualify as deductible business expenses. The same rules apply to any other members of the taxpayer's family who accompany him on such a trip.

This regulation was written some time ago, hence the masculine and feminine gender are used in the then conventional manner. Rest assured, the IRS will not allow husbands to take a tax deductible vacation along with their M.D. wives who are attending CME courses.

There are three classes of cases where the deduction for the spouse's travel expenses will be denied:

> 1. *Vacation in disguise:* where a wife or other family members are nominal employees of the taxpayer, their presence on a business trip will not have a bona fide business purpose.[14]
> 2. *Service provided that is not necessary:* wife of a doctor accompanied him on business trips, serving as his co-pilot in a plane that did not require a co-pilot.[15]
> 3. *Services at a social function:* wife attended conventions with husband and served as a hostess to other wives at receptions, or in addition does minor secretarial work.[16]

In cases involving a dispute over the spouse's travel expenses, the taxpayer bears an especially heavy burden of proving that they come within regulation §1.162-2(c). Unlike other legal situations where the individual is presumed "innocent" until the government proves otherwise, in tax law the taxpayer is entitled to a deduction only if he can prove that he meets the requirements for it as set out in law and regulation. In intrafamily matters, there is a presumption that an expenditure comes within section 262 and, therefore, is not deductible. Cases will arise in the social function category where CME sessions are held in connection with a convention, but the spouse's business contribution must be substantial to justify the deduction of his or her expenses.

The spouse's expenses will be deductible if his or her contribution to the business purpose of the taxpayer's trip is substantial, as measured by the percent of time that is devoted to it and by the type of services that are rendered. A spouse who works full-time in the taxpayer's business or profession while on the trip will meet the test.[17] Also, if the spouse has special training in the taxpayer's profession (for example, a wife who was a trained singer accompanied her singer husband and helped him rehearse[18]), his or her expenses will be deductible. To summarize, the spouse's services must be: qualitatively substantial, necessary to the taxpayer's business, and those which he could not have performed himself.

Socially related services performed, usually by a wife, can give rise to a deduction if they meet the above test. Again it is a difficult test, but it can be done. A husband whose sales business required that he develop a "very close relationship"[19] with his customers was justified in taking his wife on business trips. If the primary purpose of the trip for both spouses is to entertain company guests, all expenses for both will be deductible.[20] The socially related services of both spouses must be the means of achieving the ultimate business purpose of the taxpayer, there must be little or no time available for nonbusiness pursuits, and the spouse must spend a substantial amount of time in the performance of business services. Similar cases will arise in the context of CME trips, and where they do a deduction will be allowed for the spouse's expenses.

Foreign Travel

The same law that added the "lavish or extravagant" language to section 162 added section 274 to the IRC.[21] As to travel, this section requires an allocation of travel expense between business and nonbusiness activity for certain foreign travel. It applies to travel outside the United States, here defined to mean the fifty states and the District of Columbia. Travel to Hawaii is not restricted by section 274, but travel to Puerto Rico is. The scope of section 274 is further limited to business travel that is in excess of seven days, and where nonbusiness activity accounts for 25 percent or more of the total foreign travel days. The day of departure from the United States is not counted, but the day of return is. Therefore, if a taxpayer leaves the country on Wednesday and returns the following Wednesday, he has not been gone for 7 days and is not covered by section 274.

The operation of section 274 can best be illustrated by the two following examples. (1) A doctor flies from New York City to London for a four-day CME conference and then flies to Paris for four days of vacation. The round-trip travel expenses from New York to London are subject to allocation. The airfare is multiplied by a fraction, the numerator of which is the number of nonbusiness days; the denominator is the total number of days of the trip. In this example the fraction would be 4/8, and the amount of travel expense that could be deducted for business purposes is one-half the round-trip air fare New York to London. The round-trip air fare London to Paris is entirely personal and, therefore, not deductible. (2) A doctor travels from New York City to Rio de Janeiro for a five-day CME conference and stops in Caracas on the return for a three-day vacation. The fraction is 3/8, which is the part of the air fare that cannot be deducted as a business expense. A full deduction of the round-trip air fare Caracas to Rio de Janeiro can be taken.[22]

The allocation requirement of section 274 is in addition to those set by section 162 and the regulations thereunder. It does not make deductible an expense that is not otherwise deductible under section 162. If the taxpayer can establish that a major consideration in his decision to take a CME course abroad was not to include a vacation in addition to the CME, then the entire amount of travel expense to and from the CME site will be deductible. For example, if he can show that this was the only chance he had to take this course and that it was particularly well suited to his specialty of practice, he could deduct the entire amount.

POLICY ALTERNATIVES

Proposals have been made to change the business expense deduction law and regulations, both to liberalize and to restrict the deductibility of the expenses. It must be kept in mind that the law is the means to implement policy and that, therefore, before a change to the law can be proposed the policy objective must be defined.

Additional Expense Test

A proposal to broaden the scope of the business expense deduction advocates use of an "additional expense" test[23] to determine under present law whether an expense is business related and, therefore, deductible. This change would require a change in IRS regulations only and could be performed by the IRS. This test would divide all expenditures into three categories. The first uses the "but for" test. If a taxpayer could prove that but for a business purpose he would not have incurred the business expense, then the entire amount would be deductible, without regard to any secondary personal purposes accomplished through the expenditure. This would broaden the scope of the room and board deduction. The rationale is that any personal benefit is an incidental motivation, and rather than try to separate the mixed expenditures, the entire amount should be deductible. The second category employs the "even if" test. If a taxpayer would have incurred an expense even if there was no business purpose, then only the additional business related expense would be deductible. This would make an inroad on the "vacation in disguise" doctrine that now excludes some types of expenses.

In cases where the taxpayer cannot meet either of these tests, there would be a conclusive presumption of business expense if more than 50 percent of the expense-generating activity was due to a business purpose. That part of the mixed expense would be deductible that is equal to the percent of time that was actually spent for business purposes. This would increase the deduction that is now allowed where the expenses on nonbusiness days were greater than for business days and would allow a deduction for a part of the travel expense where the trip was primarily for nonbusiness purposes.

Tax Reform Act of 1976

The 1976 tax reform act tightens the deduction for business expenses incurred in certain foreign travel. Section 602 amends section 274 by adding a new subsection in addition to the restrictions now contained in that section. The deduction is now limited to not more than two foreign trips per year. The maximum allowable travel expense deduction is an amount equal to economy air fare to and from the CME site. To take a travel expense deduction, more than one-half the days abroad have to be devoted to a business purpose. The room and board deduction is first limited to the per diem rate for that city established for government civil servants. This includes amounts expended for lodging, meals, tips, and local transportation. To qualify for a full day deduction, the taxpayer will have to attend at least four of six hours of scheduled CME activity; a half-day deduction is available only if the taxpayer attends two of three scheduled hours of CME activity. If he attends fewer or if fewer were scheduled, there will be no deduction for room and board.

NOTES

1. Section 163, IRC; 26 U.S.C. §163. The IRS is codified in title 26 of the U.S.C. The section numbers are the same in each code. Subsequent citation will be to the IRC only.
2. Section 164.
3. Section 44(a).
4. Section 41, IRC.
5. Sections 1201, 1202, IRC.
6. 50 Cong. Rec. 3849 (1913).
7. Hearings on Tax Recommendations of the President Contained in His Message Transmitted to Congress, April 20, 1961, Before the House Committee on Ways and Means, 87th Cong., 1st Sess. 12-13 (1961).
8. 5 C.B. 171, O.D. 984 (1922).
9. §1.162-5(c)(1).
10. §1.162-5(c)(2).
11. 181 F.2d 906 (4th Cir. 1950).
12. 181 F.2d at 908.
13. The application of this regulation can be seen by contrasting two cases. The first, *Hoover v. Commissioner*, 35 T.C. 566 (1961) denied the deduction. The taxpayer, a doctor, took an eighteen-day cruise in the Mediterranean Sea, seven to ten days of which were devoted to 55 minute medical lectures followed by discussion periods. The course satisfied the doctor's CME requirement with the Academy of General Practice. The deduction was disallowed because the doctor, a busy man who often saw thirty patients a day, could have taken a similar course on land in two days for a cost of $232 (versus $1,881). The court felt he was motivated to take the cruise for personal reasons. However, in *Duncan v. Bookwalter*, 216 F.Supp. 301 (W.D. Mo. 1963), the deduction was allowed. The doctor and his wife took a four-month trip to Europe visiting alcoholism clinics similar to the one they operated in the United States. They spent most of their time visiting clinics, kept a detailed diary to substantiate their claim, and spent only a small amount of time sightseeing. The court said a taxpayer "should be

allowed reasonable latitude in determining the type of expenses incurred in connection with the research, study and etiology of this disease and its attending problems." 216 F.Supp. at 305.

14. *John A. Guglielmietti,* 35 T.C. 668 (1961).

15. *Robert H. Cowing, M.D.,* P-H Tax Ct. Mem. ¶69, 135 (1969).

16. *Sheldon v. Commissioner,* 299 F.2d 48 (7th Cir. 1962).

17. *Poletti v. Commissioner,* 330 F.2d 818 (8th Cir. 1964).

18. *John Charles Thomas,* 39 B.T.A. 1241 (1939).

19. *Warwick v. United States,* 236 F.Supp. 761 (E.D. Va. 1969).

20. *Allen J. McDonnell,* P-H Tax Ct. Mem.¶67,018 (1967).

21. PL 87-834 (1962).

22. The fraction allocation is applied to the round-trip air fare, New York to Caracas.

23. "The Additional Expense Test: Proposal to Solve Dilemma of Mixed Business and Personal Expenses," *Duke Law Journal* (August 1974): 636-637.

24. H.R. 10612.

Chapter 14
The Current Investment
in Continuing Medical Education

Lewis A. Miller

The 1907 report on continuing medical education presented by Dr. J.C. McCormack to the American Medical Association stated:[1]

> The necessity of doing something in this direction, and the magnitude of the problem, will be appreciated when it is known that a large majority of the 122,000 licensed physicians who are treating sick people every day do not attend medical meetings, and that a large percent of this element do not read research periodicals or standard literature.

Things are better by some lights. More time, money, effort, and lawmaking are being poured into CME than ever before. But still we do not know what the "something" is that we should do, nor how to define the "problem" and its "magnitude," nor how to estimate the investment and its return to physicians and their patients.

The major issues dealt with in this chapter are the following:

1. The approximate annual investment in CME on the part of physicians, hospitals, medical schools, medical associations, specialty societies, and voluntary health organizations, industry and government.
2. Methods of calculating the return on investment.
3. Public policy recommendations for the short term regarding investment in continuing medical education.

One must count on the sophisticated reader to recognize the difficulty of dealing with scanty evidence and the even greater difficulty of finding any positive conclusions to draw.

PHYSICIAN INVESTMENT

Physicians spend more time and money for their continuing education than any other professional or technical group in our society. Claims by some authors to the contrary, physicians spend more for their CME than is spent on their behalf by all others combined— including medical institutions, the government, and the pharmaceutical industry.

A survey conducted by the Iowa Medical Society and University of Iowa College of Medicine in 1973 gave a set of indicators that will be used here for estimating physician investment in CME.[2] Utilizing a random sample of 150 selected from among 2,297 members of the state medical society, the surveyors received a 79 percent response rate, which yielded a reasonable degree of statistical accuracy. There are risks in attempting to correlate responses of Iowa physicians with their counterparts in the U.S. population of 237,005 physicians engaged in patient care in 1973.[3] Nevertheless, the Iowa data can be projected for purposes of suggesting the vast investment that physicians are making in continuing education today.

The Iowa study showed that the median age of respondents was 50, that 87 percent were in private practice, and the balance in hospital or academic settings, and that the median time spent in practice (hospital or office) was ten hours per day, or 50 hours per week. (This is less than the median time reported spent by primary physicians in *Medical Economics'* 1975 surveys.)

Iowa physicians reported spending over six hours per week in CME activities. The authors add: "Since the questionnnaire unfortunately omitted the CME activities sponsored by the various specialty societies, we are inclined to believe that the true median is close to seven hours per week—*almost a full working day.*" Types of activities included journal reading, audio tapes, colleague consultation, hospital conferences, postgraduate lectures and courses, and self-assessment and home study courses.

If we speculate that the Iowa physician is typical of his colleagues across the United States, then, on the average, the American physician engaged in patient care spends at least 300 hours per year in his continuing education (the majority being spent on reading). Using the count of 237,005 such physicians, we find that they spent a grand total of 71,101,500 hours on their continuing medical education in 1973.

That staggering number of hours converts into an even more staggering amount of dollars. Here, this valuation uses the concept of "opportunity cost:" that portion of profit that is given up to do something else. In this case, one can assume that physicians are giving up their opportunity to see additional patients in exchange for continuing their education. (It must be recognized that they might instead exchange some of the time for leisure activities as well.)

In 1973, average physician income was $49,415.[4] Divided by 2,500 (assuming 50 hours a week, 50 weeks a year), the average physician net income was $20 an hour after expenses and before taxes. Multiplied by 300 hours, the opportunity cost per physician for his CME in 1973 can be placed at $6,000. This makes a grand total of $1,422,030,000 for all U.S. physicians in patient care, in private practice or on salary. (By comparison, the total cost of physician services in 1973 was estimated at $17 billion.)

The physician's out-of-pocket costs associated with CME must next be calculated, though miniscule in relation to the opportunity cost. Again, the Iowa study will be the base. On average, the responding physician spent thirty hours per year attending conferences or courses away from home or hospital; course fees averaged about $50 per day in 1973 at universities and other institutions, or $200 for four days. Travel costs were conservatively figured at $100 for those four days. Finally, $100 per year was added for journal and audio subscriptions and the purchase of a text or two. The total is $400 per physician, or projected nationally, $94,802,000 for out-of-pocket CME costs paid by physicians in 1973.

This combined total of $1,516,832,000 is an imposing figure, even if discounted for overestimation by Iowa physicians and the author. This cost later will be examined in terms of its return to the physician and to the society he serves.

HOSPITAL INVESTMENT

The Joint Commission on Accreditation of Hospitals (JCAH) has required since the mid-1960s that "the medical staff shall provide a continuing program of professional education, or give evidence of participation in such a program."[5] Some 5,000 of the nation's 7,800 hospitals have met JCAH standards.

In addition, JCAH now requires hospitals to conduct a specified number of medical audits per year, according to the number of admissions. These serve as a basis not only for quality assurance but also for continuing education. (This approximates the requirements of PSRO legislation.) Since physicians' time in CME activities includes hospital committee work, this element of CME investment is not counted again here.

One can estimate, however, costs related to full-time directors of medical education. The Association of Hospital Medical Education boasts over 600 members, most of whom spend at least 50 percent of their time on continuing education.[6] The hospital also pays fees for guest lecturers and consultants, provides committee support personnel (particularly now for quality assurance programs), and has administrative costs and floor space costs for CME programs. Most of these costs are hidden because administrators do not usually set up budgets for CME.

A reasonable minimum guesstimate in this area would be $500 per week per hospital for all such expenses, or $25,000 a year. Multiplied by 5,000 accredited hospitals, this totals $125 million. Again, this can be looked on as an opportunity cost for the third parties who pay most hospital costs. These funds could be used for direct patient care, or could represent a slight reduction in per diem charges.

MEDICAL SCHOOL INVESTMENT

The Association of American Medical Colleges has gone on record in recent years as believing that a major focus of CME should be the medical school. Even in the best of circumstances that is not yet the case, and might never be. But the role of the medical school is growing.

Medical schools accounted for 40 percent of the 4,862 courses accredited by the American Medical Association (AMA) in 1975-76 and listed in the annual supplement to the *Journal of the AMA*. The number of physician registrants at such medical school-sponsored courses grew from 73,000 in 1963-64 to 354,569 in 1973-74.[7] Only last year, a formal university group of continuing medical educators was formed.

The University of Wisconsin Department of Continuing Medical Education currently estimates it reaches 40 percent of the 5,100 practitioners in the state with some offering, and provides a "truly continuous program for less than 20 percent." The budget for this activity is $375,000 a year, of which only $125,000 is generated from fee income. Of the balance, $100,000 is from state support and $150,000 from grants and contracts.[8]

The Wisconsin budget is undoubtedly above average for the 114 medical schools across the country. At the other end of the spectrum, the new University of Nevada College of Medical Sciences spent only $2,000 — that it could account for — last year.[9]

Exclusive of physician fees but including the kinds of hidden costs for personnel, travel time, administrative costs, floor space, etc., that are often not budgeted, this author has estimated that each medical school spends an average $75,000 per year, or a total of $8.5 million, for continuing medical education. This is a small investment compared with the costs of graduate and undergraduate medical education.

MEDICAL ASSOCIATION INVESTMENT

The American Medical Association, the American Osteopathic Association (AOA), and most state and county medical societies offer CME programs at annual, quarterly, or monthly meetings. In 1973, the AMA reported state medical societies spent $1,172,085 for CME.[10] In 1975, the Massachusetts Medical Society spent over $100,000.[11] But this appears to be only the tip of the iceberg. The AMA itself has substantial costs associated with administering its Physician's Recognition Award (PRA), which 40,000 physicians received in its first three-year cycle. (Earning the PRA requires 150 credit hours of CME every three years. Organizations and institutions are accredited under this program—at last count, 1,042 institutions under 554 primary sponsors).[12] The AMA has also stepped up its own CME programs through regional institutes and more workshops at its semiannual meetings.

Twelve state medical societies—Alabama, Arizona, Florida, Kansas, Maine, Massachusetts, Minnesota, New Jersey, North Carolina, Oregon, Pennsylvania, and Vermont—have made a policy decision to require CME as a condition of membership.[13] The mechanisms for recording information and following up with reminder, or disciplinary action where necessary are costs to the medical society. The Illinois State Medical Society, without such a requirement, budgeted $93,000 in 1973 for setting up the Illinois Council on Continuing Medical Education (ICCME), and currently puts $10 of dues (or about $40,000) annually into the ICCME budget.[14] California, also not requiring CME as a condition of membership, has an extensive accreditation and coordination program under the California Medical Association. The American Osteopathic Association has a requirement for CME now that is also costly to accredit and administer.

This author's estimate is that the investment of the AMA and AOA alone total over $1,250,000. If state societies average $40,000 each, that adds up to $2,000,000. Figure another $750,000 from county and local associations for a grand total of $4 million. These figures exclude journal publication.

SPECIALTY SOCIETY INVESTMENT

Some twenty-eight of the thirty-four major national specialty societies conduct continuing education courses at their annual meetings; most of the thirty-four, such as the American College of Physicians, American College of Surgeons, and American Academy of Family Physicians, also hold local and regional CME meetings. Continuing education has long been looked on as a prime function of the specialty societies, not only for courses, but also for journals and corollary activities.

A major new activity of specialty societies is self-assessment examinations. As of early 1975, a total of thirteen societies had administered about 90,000 such tests to physicians. Nine specialty societies have full-time executives for continuing education, and six have made policy decisions to require CME for membership; though the American Academy of Family Physicians, with about 30,000 members, is the only major society implementing the policy fully.[15]

In 1973, the AMA estimated that twenty-eight specialty societies spent $10,682,860 for CME.[16] This figure rounds out to $12 million to account for the other societies. No separate estimate has been made for medical specialty boards, which are just beginning to get into CME through recertification requirements. The American Board of Family Practice is the only board that has instituted a requirement for recertification of its diplomates. But most other specialty boards have considered the question and are expected to follow suit over the next decade. Also included in this category, is the spending of specialized voluntary health agencies such as the American Heart Association, American Cancer Society, American Lung Association, and Muscular Dystrophy Association, which spend a minor part of their income on professional education each year, perhaps totaling $1 million. Folding in the costs of specialty societies, specialty boards and voluntary health agencies, this category of CME investment totals $13 million.

INDUSTRY INVESTMENT

Private enterprise, including the pharmaceutical industry, the private education industry, and the publishing industry, has made a thriving business in CME. Much of the material is provided to physicians free of charge, paid for directly or indirectly by the pharmaceutical companies, and occasionally by others in the medical supply field or in the insurance industry.

The Pharmaceutical Manufacturers Association reported in 1974 on a survey response by forty of its 115 member companies:[17]

> The total number of pieces of print material (monographs, books, etc.) in circulation by the industry . . . that serve to advance the knowledge of health professionals came to 974 nonproduct-related items . . . and 1,811 product-related items. . . . The number of films and major audiovisual items . . . amounted to 2,945 nonproduct-related items . . . and 237 product-related items. . . . The number of major symposia, conferences, meetings, or forums sponsored annually . . . amounted to 2,965 nonproduct-related and 5,779 product-related.

In testimony before the Senate Monopoly Subcommittee in April, 1976, Dr. Richard Croul, Director of the Bureau of Drugs of the Food and Drug Administration, stated that "much of the written and audiovisual teaching material supplied to the physician on all medical subjects throughout his professional career is supported by the pharmaceutical industry. This includes the vast majority of medical magazines which fill his mailbox, the clinical symposia that discuss specific drugs . . . the audio-visual teaching systems he studies in his spare time, the films and closed circuit TV tapes he sees in hospital conferences, and even the scientific exhibits and presentations by panels of experts he encounters at medical meetings."[18]

The investment by the pharmaceutical industry in all forms of promotion, including for educational program support, has been estimated at from $430 million to $1 billion in 1971, according to Milton Silverman and Dr. Phillip R. Lee, in their book, *Pills, Profits and Politics*. One estimate they quote put the education investment category at about $150 million, plus over $100 million for advertising expenditures in support of journals (which, as already noted, are the major source of the physician's continuing education.)[19] If all promotion to physicians were considered to be "education," the pharmaceutical industry expenditure would be recorded at the $1 billion level. But here the definition is restricted to spending for what is clearly labeled "education," or $150 million.

GOVERNMENT INVESTMENT

Federal and state governments are increasingly involved in continuing education. The National Institutes of Health have always made sporadic efforts to filter the results of research through to the practitioner. Traditionally, the National Library of Medicine has served as a resource. The Center for Disease Control has disseminated information to physicians on areas of communicable and chronic disease. All these groups are stepping up their activity.

The National Library of Medicine is working on an audio-visual resource program. NIH is seeking new ways to tell its stories to those involved in patient care. Confidential sources place the CME-related spending by NIH, including the Library of Medicine, at about $55 million. But even more, other federal government agencies are moving into the CME scene. Most prominent is the Bureau of Quality Assurance, responsible for administering PSRO, with a budget of close to $50 million, which is looked on by many as being directly or indirectly 100 percent related to CME.

BQA officials, writing in the *New England Journal of Medicine*, suggest that PSROs

> should serve to institutionalize the 'Bi-Cycle' concept of continuing education, in which review of patient care identifies topics for continuing education, and continuing education is evaluated through follow-up review.
>
> Each local PSRO should serve as a clearinghouse to assure the development of appropriate educational programs . . . should work closely with hospitals, medical schools, other health professional schools, specialty societies, medical societies and appropriate voluntary health associations within its area to match their educational programs with needs identified through peer review . . . [and] should work with local institutional review committees to assure that appropriate individual programs of education are available for individual practitioners.[20]

The Food and Drug Administration has become more active in CME, probably to the tune of $2 million annually, through publications and regulation of education materials sponsored by pharmaceutical companies. The FDA now has an assistant commissioner with staff to develop programs of professional education for practitioners.

The Alcohol, Drug Abuse, and Mental Health Administration, the Health Resources Administration (including Area Health Education Centers), and the Health Services Administration (including public health hospitals, Indian Health Service, emergency medical services, maternal and child health services, etc.) are all involved in CME. For example, the National Health Service Corps is setting up a continuing education network to serve its rural practice settings around the United States. These agencies, plus the Center for Disease Control, probably spend about $4 million for continuing medical education.

Finally, the Department of Defense and the Veterans Administration, both major employers of doctors, have established programs of CME (the latter including an incentive payment for participation). The Department of the Army, for instance, ran twenty-seven CME courses last year; the Navy about twenty. Total VA and Defense spending in CME is probably $1 million.

On a state level, eight states now have passed legislation that suggests or mandates CME as a requirement for relicensure. State boards of health also have been involved in providing continuing education for physicians in some states. Again guesstimating, the state CME costs are about $500,000.

The costs of bureaucracy are not easy to estimate, particularly when merged with other services. And there is no way to determine the costs of legislative bodies to investigate, deliberate, and pass laws involving CME. Overall, however, the investment in CME activities on federal and state levels is about $112 million.

INVESTMENT SUMMARY

This crude approach to estimating the current annual investment in continuing medical education totals:

Investment by

Physicians	1,516,832,000
Hospitals	125,000,000
Medical schools	8,550,000
Medical associations	4,000,000
Specialty societies, etc.	13,000,000
Industry (excluding advertising)	150,000,000
Government	112,000,000
Total investment	$1,929,382,000

Based on the reported costs for fiscal 1974, this is equivalent to about 1.5 percent of national health expenditures. It must be recognized that the bulk of the cost for continuing education, $1.4 billion, represents physician opportunity cost and would not be covered in government cost indicators. More than $400 million in direct costs would be included, however.

RETURN ON INVESTMENT

In finance, return on investment (ROI) is measured by the profit generated in relation to the capital invested; ROI generally rises as the risk rises. In continuing medical education, ROI poses a much more difficult problem. Attempts to estimate the annual investment are difficult because of the paucity of hard data. ROI is much harder to deal with since there is no agreement either on the measurement of return to be utilized or on the percentage return that might be acceptable in view of the risks taken by the investors.

The most popular measurement used now is the credit-hour measurement, though it is not truly a measure of return but one of how some of the capital has been invested. As noted, 40,000 physicians have met the AMA requirements for the Physician's Recognition Award. About 30,000 have qualified for membership in the American Academy of Family Physicians, which also requires 150 hours every three years. Others have met the requirements of the American Osteopathic Association, state medical societies and specialty societies. (Clearly there is overlap, since requirements for many societies are similar.) Therefore, one is misleading the investors in CME by using credit hours as a measurement of accomplishment. Dr. George E. Miller, a pioneer in research in medical education, and an author in this volume, recently criticized the AMA accreditation process for failing to determine which of the 4,862 offerings by AMA accredited institutions "meet the criteria for sound education." He pointed out that the Physician's Recognition Award requires a minimum of 60 out of 150 credit hours to be taken in accredited courses but permits only a limited option for nonsupervised individual work such as self-instruction, consultation, patient care review, and self-assessment. "I acknowledge that this arrangement is easier for bookkeepers," said Dr. Miller, "but I doubt that it fosters what we say we are seeking—a lifetime learner rather than a perpetual course taker."[21]

Twenty years ago, Osler Peterson's well-known study of the quality of care also challenged the validity of measuring hours. The Peterson study found that North Carolina general practitioners who averaged about fifty hours of postgraduate study per year gave a somewhat better quality of care to their patients. But some of the highest rated physicians had taken little CME, while some of the lowest rated were frequent participants. Dr. Peterson concluded that "the data do not show that postgraduate education as conducted at present influences practice greatly."[22]

It can be argued further that the credit hour system penalizes the physician with a high rating in quality of care by requiring him to put in hours of study without cause, and without reward. The American penal system, poor as it is, recognizes the value of giving time off for good behavior. The American medical system of CME credit hours fails to do this. The steady increase in the number of physicians meeting credit hour standards can in no way be regarded as evidence of incremental profit from the increasing investment in CME.

Can knowledge testing be used instead as a valid measure of return on investment? This has been the accepted standard in most education systems, including medicine. Knowledge testing is generally used as the basis for admitting, licensing, and certifying. Society tends to believe that testing scores are a reflection of the accomplishments of our public education system (witness the general concern over the recent decline in scores on the verbal college board exams). Knowledge testing certainly has more to recommend it than credit hours as a measure, because at least it estimates a qualitative factor affecting human behavior.

At present, a number of specialty societies offer self-assessment tests. The American Board of Family Practice will shortly require its first diplomates to recertify through examination, audit of office records, and completion of 150 credit hours.

Before this approach should be widely used, however, the specialty societies must develop core curricula as a basis for testing, related insofar as possible to the needs of patients who are seen by practitioners in each discipline. In some specialties, such as the surgical specialties, knowledge testing must be accompanied by skills testing, or by some evidence from a hospital tissue committee that the surgeon meets the basic requirements for the type of surgery in which he is being recertified.

Testing in itself is not so much a measure of return on CME investment as it is a measure of the status of the physician's knowledge and skills. One begins to approximate a measure of return, however, if one can analyze the gain or loss in knowledge and skills at the end of one time period as compared with the status at the beginning. For this reason, educational objectives must be determined on a specialtywide basis; testing must be correlated with these and must be administered uniformly. The incremental value in knowledge or skills then can be quantified. For example, obstetricians in the state of Iowa might move from 78 to 83 percent in their ability, on written or simulation tests, to identify accurately high risks in pregnancy before the second trimester.

If such are the educational objectives, the next logical question is: Would performance evaluation be the best measurement of return on CME investment? Many would argue yes—particularly those who strongly build their case for improving the quality of care around the medical audit. But this author questions the validity of this method of measurement at this time. Evidence to date has not demonstrated that medical audits are a successful tool in evaluating continuing education on any uniform basis, despite the efforts of PSRO to bring the two into a close relationship. Further, there are factors that interfere with physician *performance* even when a physician is demonstrably *competent* under ideal circumstances. Interference might result from poor physical facilities, inadequate paramedical assistants, or lack of patient cooperation. These factors are often not within the control of the practicing physician, nor can they be improved, as a rule, by continuing education of the physician. (Help is needed instead to educate the hospital staff and the patient.)

Performance evaluation has significant risks, too, if the performance objectives are not correctly set. Dr. Edward Rubenstein reported the results of an experiment in CME conducted by Stanford University at a nearby community hospital. Attending physicians participated in a twice weekly lecture series geared to their needs, as identified by the Stanford faculty. The effect of the lectures was then measured by quantifying certain medical activities. For example, during a lecture on urinary tract disorders, "the value of serum creatine determinations as a serial test of renal function was stressed," Dr. Rubenstein said. "The average number of such determinations per month during the nine months prior to this lecture was 116. This number increased during the subsequent nine months to 159." This is taken as evidence that "well-conceived lectures and clinical conferences can be effective learning methods."[23]

The hazard in such a method is that the measurement of performance might be inappropriate. Three years from now, it could be that serum creatinine determinations are not the tests of choice for renal function; even today, an expert from another medical school might disagree on their importance. The numerical measurement of "success" in following a rote pattern of behavior is not necessarily a measurement of the investment in continuing education. The same criticism, of course, can be applied to measurements of knowledge and skill through testing.

Statistical measurements of morbidity and mortality could be all that is left to determine a return on CME investment. After all, these are the ultimate outcome measurements of health. But they are not specific measures of physician competence related to continuing education. Environmental, social, and demographic factors play a major role in such statistics. The time lag between cause and effect is likely to be great enough to make any correlations difficult.

Where does that leave us? First, let us recognize that continuing education is a means to an end, which is the delivery of optimal patient care. Second, we have not been successful to date in defining optimal patient care. Third, we cannot easily measure the effects of education on patient care. Fourth, we do not have core curricula, or standard educational objectives by specialty, for practicing physicians. Even if we were to measure return of CME investment against intermediate objectives through testing of competence (knowledge and skills), we do not have adequate tools to perform such testing, nor do we have the evidence that widespread testing would be a valid measurement.

Suppose for the moment that these obstacles were overcome. Suppose research had demonstrated that we can relate physician competence to patient care, and that we can evaluate continuing education by testing physician competence. We are still left with the problem of deciding the value of the return we are seeking on our investment. How much is it worth to move Iowa obstetricians from a grade of 78 to 83 percent on a biennial exam? Should it be $5,000 per physician per year? $3,000? $10,000? How do we relate this investment to a payoff in improved health status of Americans? We are far from being able to deal with such questions, and I doubt that we will develop formulas of any value within this century.

Clearly, we are faced, then, with making continued investment decisions in CME at high risk and under uncertainty. *Risk* is normally associated with those situations in which probability distribution of returns can be calculated; *uncertainty* is associated with those situations in which insufficient evidence is available even to estimate a probability distribution.

In such a situation, we can only calculate our return on investment in comparative terms. We can use the opportunity cost approach, i.e., the value of an opportunity forgone, or we can use "certainty equivalents," i.e., a comparison of the unknown with a known *riskless* investment. For example, we know that $100,000 put into a U.S. Treasury bill will yield 4.5 percent and that we will receive $100,000 back at the end of three months. A friend asks us instead to invest $100,000 in his idea to develop a time machine. We are not sure whether he can ever develop it or just what it will do, but it is an exciting idea, and might just revolutionize the world. Which choice shall we make with our $100,000? The decision is highly subjective and depends on a number of factors, such as the amount of money we have, our personality (risk-taker or risk-avoider), and our fascination with the concept.

Now look at a "certainty equivalent" situation as it applies to public policy in CME investment. Let us suppose that spending $1 billion under mandated public policy would with *certainty* keep 40,000 kidney patients alive for one more year on renal dialysis. Our alternative is to spend $1 billion on the continuing education of 237,000 physicians who provide care to 200 million Americans in the course of a year. Assuming our resources are limited, would we choose the CME investment under uncertainty, or would we choose the "certainty equivalent"?

PUBLIC POLICY ISSUES

The question posed above is neither an exercise in high drama nor a lesson in investment decision theory. It is a significant and timely issue for physicians, medical schools, societies, hospitals, industry and government. In the long run, it is the public who pays for CME through medical care fees, hospital costs, drug prices, health insurance, and taxes; the public and its elected representatives must then decide the issue.

Investment in CME has passed the point of diminishing returns. The proliferation of courses, publications, audio-visuals, regulations, and requirements for participation is constant. No agency is setting uniform standards of quality, much less rationing quantity. Doctors themselves are becoming plaintive and defensive about CME. Dr. John D. Morrocco, a primary physician in Carnegie, Pa., recently wrote in a letter to the editor of *Patient Care:* "I have always been interested in keeping up-to-date in medicine, but now that I am told I *must* have so many credit hours to maintain my membership in our societies, I resent it very much." A colleague, Dr. E.R.W. Fox, of Coeur D'Alene, Idaho, added: "With the threat of compulsory CME hovering over the practicing physician, PG(postgraduate)courses are burgeoning, and some appear to be lucrative rackets. At least two brochures come in the mail each day. Where registration fees used to range from $15 to $35, now it is not uncommon for them to be $250 to $400."[24]

A task force of the Alliance for Continuing Medical Education, an ad hoc group dealing with problems of coordination and planning in CME, stated last year:

We need to recognize that there is a limit on available resources. It may be time to cut back on quantity and improve quality. To accomplish this, we need better methods to help the physician decide what his educational needs are and how to fulfill them. We need tougher methods of assessing institutions and the CME programs they provide. We need better information for the financers of CME to enable them to make hard-nosed decisions about which CME efforts to support and to what extent.[25]

Dr. Robert K. Richards, Jr., of the University of Michigan Medical School fears that

continuation of current trends, without coordination, may lead to a future in which an individual physician would be required to:
(1) document his attendance at organized CME programs for medical *and* specialty society membership as well as for state relicensure;
(2) pass a written examination periodically for recertification by his specialty board;
(3) participate in a peer review system aimed at quality assessment as a condition of his hospital's accreditation by JCAH; and
(4) participate in a regional review system aimed at cost containment to meet PSRO prerequirements.
The cost and time requirements of such an uncoordinated CME future would be substantial.[26]

The chief concern of public policy makers, given the uncertainty of return from CME investment, should be to go slow. This author's recommendations for the next three years are the following:

1. Declare a moratorium on the effectiveness of all state and federal laws and regulations that require credit hours of CME as a condition for relicensure or reimbursement;
2. Do not demand evidence of educational change resulting from PSRO or other medical audit programs (which may result, however, in improvements in the quality of care);

3. Withhold support from new state or federal proposals to fund CME until some method of establishing efficacy has been determined;
4. Avoid regulation of CME activities on state or federal level (e.g., by the Food and Drug Administration, state medical boards, or Health Systems Agencies) that would tend to freeze or change patterns of continuing education that cannot now be properly evaluated;
5. Fund research studies through quasi-public agencies such as the Institute of Medicine or the National Academy of Sciences to determine the links between CME, physician competence, and patient care;
6. Encourage the profession to set standards of care, and in turn standards of knowledge and skills, by specialty, perhaps through a coordinating body such as the Council of Medical Specialty Societies. Encourage the new Liaison Committee on Continuing Medical Education to set uniform standards for the accreditation of continuing education institutions and programs, and to coordinate continuing education offerings to reduce waste and to improve quality.

The individual physician truly bears the responsibility for his professional activity, including his ability to assimilate new facts and skills and to discard or improve traditional practices. It is his time, money and personal devotion to his profession that make CME efforts not only possible but also profitable for himself and for his patients.

This spirit of individual physician investment is best summed in the words of the historian, Bruce Catton. He wrote in his autobiography this tribute to his father, who was an educator:

> He carried with him, from his youth to the day of his death, the notion that man is born to a splendid debt; that he owes, to some force beyond the circling stars, the duty of spending himself to the uttermost for something beyond his own well being.

NOTES

1. Robert King Richards, Jr., "Current Forces Influencing Continuing Medical Education in the United States," Dissertation, University of Michigan, 1975, p. 29.
2. Richard M. Caplan, M.D., "Survey of Continuing Medical Education in Iowa," *Journal of Iowa Medical Society* 64 (April 1974): 159-166.

3. American Medical Association, *Profile of Medical Practice* (Chicago: Center for Health Services Research and Development, AMA, 1974).

4. *Ibid.*

5. "National and Local Influence on Continuing Medical Education, *Journal of the Medical Association of the State of Alabama* 42 (April 1973): 723.

6. Conversation with Norman Stearns, M.D., president, Association of Hospital Medical Education, April 1976.

7. Richards, *op. cit.,* p. 143.

8. Harrison Owen, *Continuing Medical Education: An Assessment and Recommendations* (Chicago: Office of Prevention, Control, and Education, National Heart and Lung Institute, November 1975): p. 102.

9. *Ibid.*, p.141.

10. Continuing Medical Education, Section IV," *JAMA* 226 (November 19, 1973): 957.

11. Private communication.

12. George E. Miller, M.D., *Challenges to Continuing Medical Education* (Chicago: Center for Educational Development, University of Illinois College of Medicine, January 30, 1976).

13. *Continuing Medical Education Fact Sheet* (Chicago: American Medical Association, October 1, 1975).

14. Willard Scrivner, M.D., "Medicine: The Learned and Learning Profession," Illinois Medical Journal, 143 (June 1973): 493.

15. *AMA Continuing Medical Education Newsletter* 5 (March 1974).

16. "Continuing Medical Education, Section IV,"*op. cit.*, p. 957.

17. "The Pharmaceutical Industry's Role in Physician Information and Education" (Chicago: Pharmaceutical Manufacturers' Association, May 1974).

18. "Competency in Medical Profession: A Strategy" (Rockville, Md.: Bureau of Health Manpower, Health Resources Administration, U.S. Department of Health, Education, and Welfare, 1976).

19. Milton Silverman and Philip Lee, M.D., *Pills, Profits & Politics* (Berkeley: University of California Press, 1974).

20. William Jessee, M.D. *et al.*, "PSRO: An Educational Force for Improving Quality of Care," *New England Journal of Medicine* 292, no. 13 (March 27, 1975): 668.

21. Miller, *op. cit.*

22. Richards, *op. cit.*, p. 94.

23. Edward Rubenstein, M.D., "Continuing Medical Education at Stanford: The Back-to-Medical-School Program," *Journal of Medical Education* 48 (October 1973): 911-918.

24. Herrick Peterson, "Patient Care," *Editor's Corner* (June 15, 1976).

25. "Findings and Recommendations of Six Task Forces" (Chicago: Alliance for Continuing Medical Education, January 1976).

26. Richards, *op. cit.*, p. 193.

Part V
Policy Alternatives to Mandatory CME

Chapter 15
Challenges to Continuing
Medical Education

George E. Miller

The challenge to continuing education is scarcely new. For at least twenty years those responsible for CME have been subjected to a constant barrage of exhortations to do better. They have been lifted up by the promise which accompanied the creation of the Regional Medical Programs Service and cast down by its premature demise; they have had high hopes for successive waves of new instructional technology — from television to computers — only to find their functional utility less than their technical appeal; they keep seeking some new magic to capture the attention of practitioners while lamenting that the hucksters still have the most direct and profound impact upon what those practitioners do; they have talked endlessly about new ways to meet these responsibilities but despite acknowledged shortcomings, have multiplied the offerings built upon the old models that have proved to be so unproductive. Here and there exciting innovations have certainly emerged, but it would be difficult to support any claim that the dominant character of CME has been significantly modified during these two decades.

The challenge, then, continues unabated. It is the time left to meet that challenge that is running out. There is mounting evidence of widening disenchantment with higher education in general and costly programs of professional education in particular. Among the professions whose educational systems have been targeted for incisive scrutiny, medicine is perhaps the most prominent, not only because of its high prestige, which has often been accompanied by an insensitivity to general social problems that is unacceptable to a new generation with different values, but also because a national spotlight upon the health service delivery system has revealed so many imperfections that are said to have produced declining services and mounting costs. And in a litigious age, the perceived deficiencies and experienced

dissatisfactions are being fought through in the courts rather than
worked through in thoughtful discourse.

PUBLIC ACCOUNTABILITY AND CME

Physicians and teachers are increasingly aware of public accountability for what they profess and for what they do. The Professional
Standards Review Organization legislation aims to expose and correct
inappropriate management of hospitalized patients. The Health
Maintenance Organization legislation encourages the exploration of
alternative patterns of delivering care, patterns that reward the
preservation of health rather than relief of disease (a priority medical
educators have mouthed for years without doing very much about it.)
And hovering over all is the growing threat (or promise) of national
legislation that will require periodic relicensure of practitioners to
preclude the rapid obsolescence that seems certain to accompany an
accelerating pace of advances in prevention, diagnosis, or treatment of
disease.

Physicians and teachers have long recognized the reality of that
decay in professional competence but have shunned responsibility for
assuring the public that incompetence does not occur. Practitioners
were simply offered a steadily increasing number of opportunities to
refurbish or augment old learning without monitoring the use of those
opportunities or determining whether they added up to anything more
than a random collection of unrelated experiences. With the change in
social expectation and the growing demand for accountability, the profession now seeks to stave off the looming specter of relicensing examinations by mandating participation in what is offered. At least
twelve state societies and six specialty organizations have now
established such a requirement for continued membership; eight state
boards are authorized to do so as a prerequisite for periodic relicensure and are beginning to translate that authorization into action. The
initial trickle of interest in a compulsory mode is becoming a flood. The
American Medical Association has supported this movement by
establishing the Physician's Recognition Award as a convenient
mechanism for documenting that participation in a manner acceptable
to professional associations and licensing bodies and by developing a
continuing education accreditation program as a means of assuring the
quality of the offerings.

While acknowledging the sincerity underlying these efforts, this
author has consistently opposed what has been called the "green
stamp" system of continuing education in which participation in

wholesome activities is equated with maintenance of professional competence. It seems clear that this battle has been lost. It is now our obligation and our challenge to be sure that meeting participation requirements results in improved performance by individual physicians, as well as encouragement of the efficient and economical health care delivery system that society demands. If this new mechanism proves to be no more than an unfulfilled promise, words without substance, then what will be lost could be the last opportunity to function as a profession responsive to expectations of public account ability without intolerable coercion. What must be done to achieve the goal of program effectiveness is not as clear as what must be avoided, so let us begin with the latter (which may prove offensive to some), then move cautiously and tentatively to the former (which is unlikely to please very many).

WHERE CURRENT PROGRAMS FAIL

First, we must without reservation abandon the notion that this challenge can be met by untrained personnel. At the risk of seeming ungracious, it is noted that no more than a handful of those responsible for the CME of physicians are either trained in education or thoroughly acquainted with the literature of that emerging science. This observation does not question either the dedication or the genuine concern of these individuals for bettering the learning opportunities available to those they serve, but it may provoke a reexamination of the qualifications required to carry out this task. Preparation in medicine is only one of the keys to the kingdom over which Directors of Medical Education (DMEs) preside. It unlocks the door to familiarity with program content but not to knowledge of program process. It is the *process* of continuing education that needs attention—the process of goal definition, of program planning (in contrast to event planning), of instructional method selection and implementation, of evaluation techniques and assessment procedures, and most of all of systematic investigation into the benefits as well as the costs of these educational efforts. A wise man once observed that where data are sparse, opinions are plentiful. There are few phrases that would better characterize today's continuing medical education. Until the spirit of research begins to permeate the work in this field it is no more likely to achieve the goals to which we are committed than the practice of medicine without a foundation of research in the basic and clinical sciences.

If the pattern now being established in medicine were to serve as a model, one supposes the Association for Hospital Medical Education, whose members influence the continuing education of a vast constituency of physicians, might demand as a requirement for continued membership evidence of attendance for at least fifty hours each year in accredited courses in education. But I am no more optimistic about the usefulness of such a mandate for DME's than I am about the comparable requirement for MD's. However, it *would* be desirable for such an association, in collaboration with others active in the field of continuing education, to spell out the components of competence based upon exhibited proficiency. It might even provide a model that would allow medicine itself to escape from the murky waters of time-based certification into which it is sinking.

Second, we must relinquish the view that present accreditation methods will suffice. One can only applaud the Council on Medical Education for initiating a systematic method of looking at institutional organization and staffing for continuing education, for it was badly needed. A recent publication indicated that 85 medical schools, 109 specialty societies, 6 voluntary health associations, 11 state medical societies, 29 hospitals, and 42 other organizations have been accredited directly by the council, and an additional 293 institutions have won accreditation through the 40 state medical societies approved for this purpose. During 1975 these agencies generated 4,862 continuing education courses in 1,042 institutions under 554 primary sponsors.

In the face of such an impressive quantitative record the question of why this will not suffice might reasonably be raised. The only possible response relates to qualitative aspects of the procedure. For, like the accreditation of basic and graduate programs, the assessment of CME addresses primarily facilities and resources rather than the educational process. And like the educational programs themselves, accreditation teams seem dominated by individuals qualified in medicine rather than pedagogy. The AMA effort has successfully focused attention on the important support mechanisms without which continuing education cannot flourish. Having made that point, the same systematic attention must now be directed to determining which of those 4,862 offerings meet the criteria for sound education. The few data presently available give little reason for satisfaction with present educational practices. It is these practices, not the resources and facilities which support them, that must change if the challenge of the future is to be met and the time exposure principle for continuing education is to have any hope of real meaning.

Third, we must abandon the belief that a hospital setting is the best site for continuing medical education. It is one site, it might even be an important site, but since it is the least frequent site for provider/consumer transactions about health and illness, hospital-based CME almost inevitably takes on the flavor of cure rather than care, illness rather than health, intervention rather than support — problems that can be dealt with rather than problems that must be lived with. In these dichotomous phrases it is the second member of the pairs rather than the first that society seems to be asking us to address.

Fourth, we must give up the fiction that episodic encounters will add up to a meaningful program of personal continuing education. No matter how carefully an individual program is planned or conducted it has little hope of being more than an interlude unless it is integrated into the professional life of the participant. Although not all planners try to capitalize upon the principle of detachment as openly as some of the entrepreneurs whose colorful brochures appear to have been developed by travel agents rather than educators, nonetheless the tone of much that masquerades as CME is one of escape from, rather than immersion in, the work of medicine.

Certainly an objective observer looking at the Physician's Recognition Award might understandably conclude that the best of continuing education was to be found on the edge of professional life rather than at its heart. Category one activities (i.e., those with "accredited sponsorship," which means, for the most part, courses) not only *can* be used to meet the full requirement of 150 credit hours but *must* be used for at least 60. Category five activities (i.e., nonsupervised individual work such as self-instruction, consultation, patient care review, self-assessment) are not only *optional* but can be employed to fulfill *only* a limited portion of the credit requirement. Such criteria would appear to encourage the kind of episodic continuing education that is now so prominent and to discourage the continuity that is so badly needed. This arrangement is easier for bookkeepers, but it does not foster what should be the goal — a lifetime learner rather than a perpetual course taker. But this is not a problem for CME alone; it is one that can be found at every level of the educational continuum. Even a graduate school dean in a moment of despair over courses and credits was once heard to say that "academic red tape threatens to stifle the spirit of higher education."

Finally, we must abandon the position that a significant program of continuing education can be carried out in the absence of clearly defined responsibility and authority. What is everybody's business is nobody's business. Yet that is precisely where medicine finds itself as the pressures are mounting for public assurance that individual practitioners will maintain continuing competence to provide the entire population with required health services, at a price society can afford.

It is naive to expect that this goal will be achieved if the task is left to the now accredited 552 primary sponsors of the 1,042 institutional programs (supplemented by innumerable applicants awaiting accreditation) if they continue to operate independently, without a general plan or coordinated effort. A system is what is needed.

THE CHANGES THAT ARE DEMANDED

And thus it is necessary to move from what must be avoided to what logic suggests is demanded. That consideration might begin with the prophetic words Ward Darley wrote about continuing education just fifteen years ago:[1]

> A challenge is posed for educational pioneering and innovation of a kind never before attempted. Casual methods, superficial and patronizing instruction or discursive filibustering can have no place in an effective effort of this kind.
>
> The need is for: (1) educational enterprise in the real sense of the term—continuing, comprehensive educational programs which effectively interpret the changing body of medical knowledge in a manner appropriate for mature members of a learned profession; (2) a method of transmission or delivery which meets the practical considerations of a physician's everyday situation; and (3) an effort that is protected against exploitation from any quarter....
>
> With these thoughts and situations in mind this presentation is made to propose the establishment of a National Academy of Continuing Medical Education.

Those words triggered action. In May 1961 the Board of Trustees of the American Medical Association, with seven cosponsoring professional organizations, appointed a joint study committee to "spell out the dimensions of a program of continuing medical education." The result of that work was a 1962 report by the study director, Bernard Dryer, entitled "Lifetime Learning for Physicians"[2] in which these paragraphs will be found:

> A partnership among the proven abilities of several of our major medical resources will give strength to all which none

can possess separately. Although such alliances and federations must ultimately be controlled . . . by individual personal decisions and local community requirements the administrative cohesion must first occur at the national level. . . .

The opportunity can be realized with relative swiftness by setting it upon this tripod: (a) a reexamination of our ideas as to what constitutes the true continuing education of a physician; (b) the translation of these ideas into an administrative partnership of our best available teaching resources; (c) the wide utilization of imaginative tools offered by modern technology to reinforce the teaching/learning process.

Like the creation of a new medical school and teaching hospital this plan will require the formation of a task force which will provide continuity of policy, planning, coordination, and administration, for this proposal is in a sense the design for a nationwide university without walls.

It is sad to recall that the coalition of sponsoring organizations disbanded following publication of the report, each to pursue an independent path. Only the American Medical Association made any substantial attempt to translate Dryer's words into an action program. The National Plan for Continuing Education, which was launched in 1963 under the direction of Patrick Storey, ran an exciting and innovative course for three short years. The report of that adventure, by Storey, Williamson, and Castle[3] is another significant landmark in the history of CME, one which can offer important guidelines to a profession which might now, ten years later, be more receptive to what they attempted. Looking back over what had been achieved and what remained to be done, the authors said:

> . . . if the concept is adopted that real progress in continuing medical education can be made only when the problems of medical care itself are carefully identified, then it follows that physicians themselves must be given the opportunity to share in the diagnostic process that will disclose the dimensions of the problem. . . .
>
> The problems of medical care and the problems of continuing medical education are not separable. . . .
>
> There is no doubt that the task is almost overwhelming in the amount of work yet to be done, but that is why national resources must be used.

And thus the new challenges have already been addressed by esteemed colleagues for whose proposals the world of medicine was not yet ready. It may still be unready. For if such visions are to become reality both those who sponsor and those who seek continuing education will have to give up some treasured notions about what it is and how it needs to be organized. We might not have the statesmen required to establish a system of institutions and *lifetime registration* of *every* practitioner in an individualized CME program addressed to the maintenance of defined competence, not merely the accumulation of academic credits; but we must seek them — and quickly.

In quantitative terms the problem is not insurmountable. If for purposes of identifying the necessary resources we accept the current standard of fifty hours of continuing education annually for each of the roughly 350,000 active practitioners, that comes to only 8,750 man years each year. This is less than that required annually for each entering class of medical students, a requirement that is met by a system of 110 medical schools, in contrast to ten times as many organizations which now provide less continuing education for fewer full-time students. It takes no giant intellect to recognize that the immense investment that is now scattered could be used more efficiently and more productively if random activities were replaced by systematic efforts. The question, of course, will be who runs the system.

This author would be reluctant to assign that responsibility to any one of the major groups which now claims it — the medical schools, the hospitals, the professional societies — for they have accumulated what can only be described as a long history of failure in this field. Darley suggested a national academy. Why not regional consortia, independently chartered as educational institutions, supported by both tuition fees and public and private funds, guided by a board of directors representing all interested groups (including consumers), and staffed by a faculty that accepts research into continuing education as well as delivery of continuing education as the responsibilities for which they would be held accountable. Such specification should lay to rest any possibility of interpreting this as a suggestion to resurrect the postgraduate schools, which never met such rigorous demands. These newer academies would differ from any past organization in having a constituency of continuously registered lifetime learners rather than occasionally registered episodic students. If mandatory CME is here, then let the mandate be one which assures both a continuity of relationship with a single educational organization and individualized education in the interest of maintaining professional competence, rather than encouraging interrupted relationships with a variety of institutions in the interest of fulfilling a credit requirement.

Despite the praiseworthy efforts of many individuals during the last ten years, it is difficult to avoid the uncomfortable feeling that we have been in the thick of thin things, to use Dorothy Parker's colorful phrase. Unless we are willing to risk a fundamental change in the orientation and organization of CME, there is probably little reason to hope that the future will be very different from the past.

It may be useful to end this essay with the words of John Gardner,[4] who wrote not many years ago:

> Today we can't afford not to take chances. I am always puzzled by people who talk as though the advocates of change [were] just inventing ways to disturb the peace in what would otherwise be a tranquil community. We are not seeking change for the sheer fun of it. We must change to meet the challenge of altered circumstances. Change will occur whether we like it or not. It will either change in a good and healthy direction or change in a bad and regrettable direction. There is no tranquility for us.
>
> We can choose not to accept the challenge, of course, but then we shall fall very rapidly into the ranks of the museum nations, and tourists from more vigorous lands will come from afar to marvel at our quaint ways.

NOTES

1. Ward Darley and Arthur S. Cain, "A Proposal for a National Academy of Continuing Medical Education," *Journal of Medical Education* 36 (January 1961): 33-37.

2. Bernard V. Dryer, "Lifetime Learning for Physicians," *Journal of Medical Education*, 37 (Supplement to June 1962).

3. Patrick B. Storey, John W. Williamson, and C. Hilmon Castle, *Continuing Medical Education, A New Emphasis* (Chicago: American Medical Association, 1968).

4. John W. Gardner, *No Easy Victories* (New York: Harper and Row, 1968).

Chapter 16
Can CME Be Made Part of a Medical Education Continuum?

John A. D. Cooper

The title of this chapter suggests that there is some question about whether continuing medical education is now an integral part of the educational and training continuum for physicians. There is good reason for such doubt. Continuing medical education has not actually developed within the mainstream of medical education. Although the Voland report to the American Medical Association (AMA),[1] the Dryer report,[2] the Coggeshall report,[3] and the Millis report[4] all recommended that medical schools assume institutional responsibility for CME, the schools have not generally seized the opportunity. This response has occurred despite the fact that their faculties might be considered the logical resources of leadership and talent for this phase in the continuum of the education and training of physicians.

Why has this occurred? In part because medical schools do not give high priority to responsibilities for educating their students after they have acquired the MD degree or completed specialty training in affiliated teaching hospitals. It has also been due to the increasing competition for funding. The pressures of larger medical school classes, mounting demands for the education and training of other health professionals, and expanded patient care responsibilities have taxed the ever less adequate financial and human resources of the academic medical centers. Continuing medical education has not fared well under this difficult set of circumstances. CME has usually been assigned to an organizational unit that has not shared in the esteem and institutional financing given to other medical school programs. It has had to depend largely on the entrepreneurial capabilities of the director, who has been required to float his tub on its own financial bottom.

Another reason that CME has not been incorporated into the educational continuum is the increasing uncertainty about whether, in its traditional form, it can help physicians achieve a high level of performance. This questioning of a commonly held article of faith is the consequence of the growing body of evidence that conventional approaches to continuing education, while giving the appearance of improving knowledge and performance, really have little impact on the quality of the physician's practice. In fact, some claim that such approaches might actually lower the quality of the medical services provided.[5] Thus, serious doubts are being raised if the time and effort expended on the current modes of CME are really worthwhile in comparison with the other activities that they displace. The lack of recognition of CME faculty through academic appointments, promotion, or tenure is an example of the low regard in which the department is held.

IS CME EFFECTIVE?

Despite studies demonstrating their lack of effectiveness, first reported by Youmans in 1935,[6] and subsequently verified by other careful workers,[7,8,9] the number of continuing education courses expands each year. The American Medical Association continues to accredit courses, and, increasingly, state medical societies and specialty groups are moving to mandate member participation. It has even been suggested that the federal government require periodic relicensure of physicians and dictate continuing education requirements to the states.[10] Everyone seems anxious to admire the emperor's new clothes. Few are willing to confront the naked fact that CME courses, in most instances, do not improve the provision of patient services by physicians.

Indeed, the momentum is in the opposite direction. Over the past few years, the AMA has delegated to forty-eight state medical associations the authority to accredit agencies providing CME within their states. This means that in at least these states the medical association is now empowered to approve for CME credit any institution or organization it chooses. The AMA issues a Physician's Recognition Award to those who attend a minimum of 150 hours of CME education over a three-year period in these accredited courses. Committee reports and floor debates in both the Michigan and Ohio Legislatures indicate that policy makers believe that continuing education requirements will decrease the rate of malpractice litigation, again without evidence to support the belief. At present, three states require that a physician enroll in a specified number of courses to maintain his license (Kansas, Maryland, and New Mexico). In seven additional states, the licensing boards have been empowered to establish continuing education requirements without specification of the number of hours (California, Illinois, Kentucky, Michigan, Ohio, Washington, and Wisconsin). The state medical societies in 14 states have set similar requirements for membership (Alabama, Arizona, Florida, Kansas, Maine, Massachusetts, Minnesota, Montana, New Jersey, New York, North Carolina, Oregon, Pennsylvania, and Vermont). The American Academy of Family Practice requires 150 hours of CME in each three-year period to maintain certification as a family physician.

The American Board of Internal Medicine has offered a voluntary recertification examination and the American Boards of Surgery and Pediatrics are considering similar programs. Several boards are thinking of mandating recertification for future diplomates, exempting those presently certified under a grandfather clause.

There is no question that both the public and private sectors share a legitimate concern with improving the quality of medical care. The current era of consumerism and accountability has brought increased pressure to require physicians to demonstrate their continuing competence to practice medicine. The escalation in malpractice awards has been offered as evidence of the failure of physicians to maintain their professional competence. Congress has responded by legislating programs designed to assure quality of care through the establishment of Professional Standards Review Organizations and by threatening even greater federal intervention.

CAN CME IMPROVE QUALITY OF CARE?

Clearly the goal of improving the quality of medical practice is proper and must be addressed. As members of a learned profession, physicians must not only master a substantial body of knowledge and develop skills during a long and arduous period of formal education, but they must also continue to learn for the entire period of their professional life. But approaches dictated by subjective impressions rather than by thoughtful and objective consideration of how to meet this goal effectively will waste valuable resources without producing the desired outcome. Professional organizations and public officials now racing to leap aboard the continuing education bandwagon must better understand how continuing education can be designed to have a more meaningful impact on medical practice.

We cannot assume that merely making new information more appealing and more convenient, whether by programmed instruction, conferences, seminars, audiotapes, television, etc., is a response to the problem. There must be a willingness and even enthusiasm for evaluating the impact of any approach on the ultimate aim of continued learning, to improve the quality of medical services provided by a physician through expansion of his knowledge, the sharpening of his diagnostic acumen, and the continual development of his professional skills. As George Miller observed, too often the objectives have been identified as giving the overworked practitioner an opportunity "to dip into the treasures the teacher can provide for him. And on those rare occasions when we press him, he demonstrates that he can recall verbatim (or at least in reasonable facsimile) the information he has sampled, then we are very pleased, particularly if he also reports that he has enjoyed both the dose and the vehicle."[11]

Lectures, largely abandoned by clinical departments in the undergraduate medical education program, are the mainstay of CME. This instrument is even less appropriate for mature physicians who are more oriented toward learning by doing and less interested in being a passive recipient of information in the classroom setting. Approaches must be modified if they are to be effective.

IMPROVING PHYSICIAN HABITS

Intrinsic incentives do not always provide optimal motivation for the physician to improve his practice habits. However, it is known that physicians can change their methods of practice if external incentives are provided. Lemcke[12] found that the medical audit produced a dramatic fall in the number of unjustified operations in a community hospital with no accompanying CME program. Williamson et al.[13] found that the identification of practice shortcomings, devising a program of education to overcome these faults, and then monitoring the effect of the educational program on practice, was an effective way to improve the quality of medical service. This concept was validated and expanded by Brown and Uhl at Chestnut Hill Hospital in Pennsylvania.[14] (See Chapter 2.)

Priorities for development of performance criteria are established by identifying the diseases that cause the greatest portion of disability in the patients seen by the physician. Performance criteria can be modified as new knowledge becomes available and from information collected on the effectiveness of the performance criteria in affecting the patient's outcome. The comparison of actual physician performance against the performance criteria identifies deficiencies in physician knowledge, actions or behavior and serves as the basis for educational program objectives. Reauditing of physician performance after the corrective action provides the means to evaluate the success of the intervention. The audit seems to be essential in maintaining the physician's interest in the program. The quality assurance program in PSROs can furnish the framework on which performance criteria and audit or performance can be established.

MEDICAL SCHOOL FACULTIES AND CME

Medical school faculties can make important contributions to this method of continuing education by working with the practicing physicians in developing the performance criteria and by providing the educational programs designed to correct the practice deficiencies identified through the audits. This would be a more effective use of faculty time than their involvement in a conference on "What's New In Endocrinology," or "Modern Treatment of Urinary Tract Disease."

Faculty members can also contribute to CME by motivating young physicians to accept the concept of a lifetime of learning. One of the stated objectives of undergraduate medical education is to help the student establish essential habits of continuing self-education. Changes in the medical curriculum, which give the student more individual responsibility for learning under the guidance of the faculty rather than being a passive recipient of knowledge poured forth in lectures, attempt to stimulate a scholarly attitude. This stimulus continues in the good programs of graduate medical education. However, there is evidence that we have not been completely successful in meeting our educational goals. What else can be done? We can provide a better opportunity for the student to develop a rational, objective method, one that will enable him, after he leaves the medical school and teaching hospital environment, to appraise his own deficiencies and those of other health professionals with whom he is involved. One approach that has been proposed by the AAMC is to stimulate student-operated, and faculty-supervised programs that will assess the quality of the patient care in which the students are involved. In this way students can obtain a better appreciation and understanding of the need to develop a formal method of self-appraisal. This can provide an important stimulus to continued learning and be helpful in the self-diagnosis of learning needs. A few schools have introduced such programs. Their experiences are described in a special series of articles in the December 1975 *Journal of Medical Education.*

THE INFORMATION OVERLOAD

We should also help the student develop a practical method for gathering and assessing new information of importance to his practice. The current information overload is a deterrent to continued learning. The multiple approaches commonly adopted by the student as he progresses through his education do not give him an adequate basis to sort out and retrieve new knowledge and information as he practices medicine. Although there is no objective evidence to support the view, more attention to these aspects of medical education would probably reinforce other measures that encourage the physician to become a lifetime learner.

It is commonly assumed that practitioners need more information. As George Miller put it ten years ago: ". . .the cries of despair are mounting as the gap allegedly widens between the explosive growth of new knowledge and its application at the bedside." Miller further points out that "the exquisite elaborations of contemporary investigation are generally of major significance in the case of a relatively few patients. In an eager dissemination of new information, we seem most often to be working at the upper extremity of an S-shaped curve where immense instructional investment is likely to result in a very small increment in the quality of patient care."[15] The greatest contribution to improvement in the quality of medical services can be achieved by getting the physician to apply the information he already possesses.

In any successful program of CME, the medical school faculties will play an important role. They will be responsible both for the cultivation of learning habits in physicians and for the development of educational programs geared to correct identifiable deficiencies. But mandatory programs of CME could place too great a burden on the medical school faculties. For example, if all 350,000 physicians in the United States were required to obtain fifty hours of CME per year, 17,500,000 individual contact hours would be required. The average medical school supplies 1,000 contact hours for 400 enrolled students, or 400,000 individual contact hours per year. Thus, the increased load for fifty mandated hours of CME would be equivalent to providing faculty for forty additional medical schools. Moreover, this estimate only considers the time required for direct educational activities, excluding the time which would be required to audit and reaudit the physician's performance to define deficiencies and determine improvement. If CME requirements were imposed utilizing such a result-oriented method, the commitment of time and personnel would be mammoth.

If CME is closely coupled to the assessment of the deficiencies of physicians against performance criteria for the care of their own patients, it can become an important part of the continuum of education and training of the physician. If the traditional approaches are maintained, continuing education should probably be confined to exciting and enchanting locations. In this case, the claim made in a travel folder received by physicians is probably correct: "The concept of continuing one's professional education during relaxed travel abroad has met with gratifying acceptance."

NOTES

1. D.D.Voland, "Preview of Principal Findings of AMA Survey of Post- graduate Medical Education;" *JAMA* 155 (1954): 389-392.
2. B.V. Dryer, "Lifetime Learning for Physicians: A Report from the Joint Study Committee in Continuing Medical Education," *Journal of Medical Education* 37 (part 2) (June 1962): 1-34.
3. L.T. Coggeshall, *Planning for Medical Progress Through Education* (Evanston, Illinois: Association of American Medical Colleges, 1965).
4. J.S. Millis, Chairman, *The Graduate Education of Physicians.* The Report of the Citizens' Commission on Graduate Medical Education. (Chicago: American Medical Association; 1966).
5. G.N. Libby *et al.,* "Help Stamp Out Mandatory Continuing Education," *JAMA* 233 (1975): 797-799.
6. J.B.Youmans, "Experience with a Postgraduate Course for Practitioners: Evaluation of Results," *Journal of the Association of American Colleges* 10 (1935): 154-173.
7. O.L. Peterson *et al,* "An Analytic Study of North Carolina General Practice," *Journal of Medical Education* 31 (Part II) (1956): 1-165.
8. J.W. Williamson *et al,* "Continuing Education and Patient Care Research: Physician Response to Screening Test Results," *JAMA* 201 (1967): 938-942.
9. C.E. Lewis and R.S. Hassanein, "Continuing Medical Education— An Epidemiologic Evaluation," *New England Journal of Medicine* 282 (1970): 254-259.
10. S. 3885, 93d Congress, 2d Session, 1974.
11. G.E. Miller, "Continuing Education for What?" *Journal of Medical Education* 42 (1967): 320-326.

12. P.A. Lemcke, "Medical Auditing by Scientific Methods Illustrated by Major Female Pelvic Surgery," *JAMA* 162 (1956): 646-656.

13. Williamson *et al., op. cit.*

14. C.R. Brown, Jr., and H.S.M. Uhl, "Mandatory Continuing Education—Sense or Nonsense?" *JAMA* 213 (1970): 1660-1668.

15. Miller, *op. cit.*

Chapter 17
Future Role of the Medical School, Community Hospital, and Medical Society in Continuing Medical Education

Philip R. Manning

INTRODUCTION

Effective continuing medical education based on identification of needs in a practice setting will affect all facets of the medical profession. For this reason, a broad participation of physicians and their societies in association with other health professionals and their societies is necessary.

In this chapter I have attempted to outline appropriate roles for various professional organizations and societies. Emphasis is on the roles of medical schools, community hospitals and medical societies and the role of the proper use of the computer as a tool in continuing education.

The definition of continuing education is important. While no one argues over the concept of life-long learning, traditional classroom continuing education has been under fire as being ineffective in improving health care. The pioneering concepts and work of Miller,[1] Williamson,[2,3,4] Gonnella,[5] Brown,[6] Peterson,[7] and others have broadened the scope of continuing education to include actual problems in patient care. This concept, although well-founded, has not been universally adopted and the words "continuing education" still conjure up the image of an audience passively listening to an expert. If progress is to be made in continuing education a broad concept must supplement the narrow concept of transmission of information in a classroom or by audiovisual devices. *Continuing medical education must be built into the systems of health care delivery.*

Application of existing computer technology makes possible the implementation of the concept of patient care, problem-linked continuing education. It might well be that the computer will prove essential to the future development of practice-based continuing education.

The following discussion elaborates on five proposals for policy recommendations that demand action by the profession, the medical schools, the medical societies and the specialty societies.

FIVE POLICY RECOMMENDATIONS

1. Because of the essential resources of faculty, medical schools cannot escape a central role in CME. This central role should be accepted formally.

2. To place legislative decisions on continuing education on sounder ground, research and development centers in continuing education and quality assurance should be established in eight to ten medical schools in cooperation with county and state medical societies.

3. To establish an educational continuum, medical schools should alter their educational methodologies to include experience with the concepts and techniques of practice-based continuing education.

4. Several community hospitals in cooperation with medical schools, county, state and specialty societies should work with appropriate computer resource organizations to perform a study to evaluate patient care oriented management information systems from the standpoint of efficiency, reliability, and cost effectiveness. Following this, if considered feasible and cost effective, several demonstration models of in-hospital computerized systems should be established. The following characteristics should be incorporated into the system.[8] It should:

- provide elements of logic, memory, coordination, and feedback;
- provide support for physicians' workups and therapy plans;
- provide concurrent data relative to diagnosis therapy, discharge records, etc.;
- provide necessary fiscal information with respect to pharmacy, laboratory, and other departments;
- provide feedback for quality of care, continuing medical education, and patient education; and
- assure confidentiality.

5. Each state society should organize a committee or federation to develop and monitor state plans for CME. The committee would consist of representatives from several state groups such as the state society, specialty organizations, state board of medical examiners,

medical schools, and hospital associations. The state committee will interface with the Liaison Committee on Continuing Medical Education (LCCME).

ROLE OF MEDICAL SCHOOLS

General Roles

Until quite recently a majority of medical schools, considering themselves overcommitted in terms of teaching undergraduates and graduates, doing research, and conducting medical practice, have given continuing education low priority. As concern in quality assurance, relicensure, recertification, and other legislative and social pressures has developed, many medical schools have become more actively involved.

Despite the fact that many, if not most, medical schools have attempted to avoid significant formal involvement in CME, medical schools have actually played a central role in almost all existing continuing education programs. Regardless of what organization or society is sponsoring an educational experience, the faculty is almost entirely acquired from medical schools. Because of the very significant involvement of medical school faculty in all types of continuing education, medical schools will continue to play a central role in continuing education, formally or informally, whether they wish to do so or not.

Medical schools can most effectively link experience in the new continuing education with students and house staff to provide the base for a true educational continuum designed to help the physician in his quest to offer ever-improving health care. It is, therefore, logical for medical schools to assume greater formal responsibility for continuing education.

Medical schools should include the field of continuing education as a subject for their traditional roles of research and teaching. Despite the excellent breakthroughs that have been achieved, more research is required to devise appropriate, automatic, and "noninvasive" techniques of determining true educational and organizational needs as well as techniques of determining the proper response to the needs. The methodologies of continuing education need be taught to the profession.

Legislators are beginning to include in the law requirements for CME. It is essential that experiments and trials which determine the most effective methodologies of continuing education be carried out before more legislation is created. This research and development can best be implemented by the establishment of continuing education research and development centers in eight to ten medical schools in cooperation with county, state, and national medical societies.

Specific Services to Various Groups

In addition to being a general and central resource of continuing education, medical schools must serve various groups.

Undergraduate Students

The concept of a continuum in education has received verbal support from educators around the world for centuries. Few disagree with Malcolm Knowles in this definition of education ". . . it is no longer functional to define education as a process of transmitting what is known; it must now be defined as a life-long process of discovering what is not known."[9]

From the operational aspects of medical school teaching and learning, however, the concept of the continuum has been, in most cases, lip service to a self-evident truth. Medical students in their orientation meeting on opening day of the freshman year are told that they are entering a profession which requires life-long learning. They are reminded of this again at graduation. In between, in almost all of the medical schools, they receive an experience based on transmittal of information and heavy reliance on the ability to recall facts. They receive little instruction on techniques, concepts and organizational principles which will allow them to continue their education once they have graduated. They might hear in a lecture about the techniques of quality assurance, techniques which allow for the determination of specific needs, but they usually do not see their faculty operate in this setting. They might hear about the concepts of procedural and educational audits of the medical record, but they seldom are given the opportunity of developing their education around the material derived from audit. They are seldom, if ever, taught the importance of the physician organizing his office so it becomes the center for his own continuing education. Without a change in the direction of clinical teaching of medical students toward concepts of audit and quality assurance followed by appropriate action, continuing education will remain chiefly a classroom activity. The methodologies of continuing education need to be taught by precept and example to medical students.

Faculty

In the last several years most medical schools, through practice plans, have begun to enlarge their involvement in patient care. This involvement offers a golden opportunity for medical school faculties to develop and experiment with practice models that will have built-in methods for the identification of educational and organizational needs through the audit of process and outcomes. It thus offers the faculty the opportunity to develop responses to problems and deficits in their own patient care. It is essential that the material derived from faculty audit data be utilized in the education of the faculty itself and by the faculty in the education of medical students and house staff.

House Staff

A university teaching service is potentially an excellent environment to provide residents with actual experience in the new continuing education, i.e., experience in audit and the use of audit in determining educational and attitudinal needs and organizational problems. An auditable chart, such as the problem-oriented record, is an essential part of a teaching service. The auditable record is, however, simply a tool; and unless proper audit procedures and proper response to audit occur, little or no education or improvement in patient care can be expected to take place. The opportunity for residents to audit charts of their fellow residents is an important part of graduate training.

Certain services in university hospitals provide ideal opportunities for the educational use of data collected on the performance of specific residents. These opportunities are usually underdeveloped. For example, how many intensive care units determine how often complications with venous catheterization occur in the unit? How many hemorrhages, infections, damage to adjacent structures and pulmonary emboli occur after catheterization by a particular resident? How does this compare with others? How many complications occur with intubation? How often is the procedure done by a particular resident followed by atelectasis? If the statistics show that some residents are having poorer results than others, it seems mandatory that these residents receive appropriate education and practice on the specific procedures.

If the risk in classroom teaching is that the material may be useless and given at an inappropriate time, the risk of basing education around real and specific problems as determined by medical audit is that it may be considered threatening and even punitive. As we begin to approach sensitive and personal areas in education, medical school faculties might need to improve methods of teaching from specific information without inhibiting learning or dampening the residents' zest for learning. Decreasing enthusiam in the process of learning from actual individualized performance data will lessen the likelihood that the system will be carried out efficiently in the practice setting.

Practicing Physician

Traditional postgraduate courses offered to the practicing physician continue to be the major response of most medical schools to the need for CME. Despite the unpopularity of these courses with most planners and experimentors in the field of continuing education, the experience has not been entirely unsatisfactory. As measured by pre- and post-testing, classroom courses for the physician can result in factual learning.[10,11] Good classroom courses can heighten the enthusiam and zest of the physician for his practice. Finally, classroom courses can help the physician gain an overview of significant developments in a specific field. Some postgraduate courses are organized to address particular problems in patient management. However, the usual postgraduate course cannot be expected to offer the kind of experience which will allow for direct and measurable improvement in patient care.[12] Medical schools must seek additional methods by which they can help the physician with his hospital and office practice.

Medical School Linkage with Community Hospital

An effective way of helping the practitioner in hospital practice is to develop a link between medical schools and community hospitals. One such linkage is taking place at the University of Southern California School of Medicine. The Postgraduate Division has started to work with community hospitals that wish to become intramural teaching centers for their professional staffs. The medical school response to community hospitals takes into account the significant limitation imposed by an already overworked faculty. There are five components in the Community Hospital Plan.

First, there is an educational development team consisting of three individuals—an educational psychologist, a nurse, and a school teacher. Their function is to help the professional staff develop a meaningful procedural and educational audit and from this information develop a statement of educational and organizational needs. In many cases, resources within the community hospital can solve the particular problems. When they cannot, a faculty response to the problem is developed. The response could be an in-person visit of an appropriate faculty member to answer specific questions about the identified needs. In some cases, communication may be by telephone in response to the questions determined by audit via a speakerphone to a group of involved physicians at the hospital. On occasion, an audiovisual response is provided. All these methods tend to take less time than the previous hospital staff lectures and noon conferences that our faculty had been providing. The second component of the Hospital Network is a multidisciplinary advisory council. This group, which consists of physicians, nurses, hospital administrators, biomedical engineers, and clinical pharmacists is available to network members to consult, as a team, on a problem which reasonably may have a multidisciplinary solution. Interestingly enough, the service is seldom called upon by the community hospitals. When it has been called upon, however, it is interesting to note that in preparing the questions for the multidisciplinary council to respond to, individuals in the community hospital may meet and settle the problem to their satisfaction before the council meeting. In this circumstance, the multidisciplinary council can act as a sounding board for the proposed plan. The third component of the school's contributions consists of seminars on techniques of quality assurance and continuing education for the individuals responsible for organizing the hospital program. The fourth component is the delivery of information by audio-visual responses and better use of the library. Finally, individual physicians and nurses whose hospitals belong to the Community Hospital Network are encouraged to attend regularly scheduled on-campus programs at a significant reduction in tuition. There is an attempt to utilize the data collected in the hospital to formulate educational goals for our on-campus classroom courses.

Our experience with the Community Hospital Network, as with the experience of others, indicates that in most cases attitudinal and organizational barriers are a greater problem than actual deficits in knowledge. This, in part, may be due to the somewhat simplistic state of the art of criteria setting and audit procedures. However, at the current level of sophistication the audit provides useful material that may be used to alter organizational approaches in the community. Frequently, the audit procedure leads to discussion among the physicians in the community hospital which leads to the formulation of numerous questions which require an expert opinion. This part of the procedure needs to be further developed and it is here that university faculty members are playing a significant role.

Office Practice

The services provided at the University of Wisconsin College of Medicine by Meyer and Sivertson[13,14] and the techniques developed by Hamaty[15] in West Virginia serve as a take-off point for further involvement of medical schools in CME based on experience within the physician's office. Another interesting model has been established by Dr. Warren Williams,[16] a family practitioner in the Denver area who has developed his office as a base for his continuing education. Dr. Williams has devised a procedural audit that is carried out by his nonphysician staff. He has utilized the problem-oriented record and developed a file system which allows him to identify the problems that he is seeing. He organizes office grand rounds during which time his office will be closed and an expert from the medical school faculty will review specific problems using his medical record as a basis for instruction. The formulation of problem lists, the evolution of diagnostic and therapeutic plans and monitoring plans are discussed in detail. This type of education is very specific to patient care and provides Dr. Williams with individualized instruction. It is unlikely that medical schools could develop this specific type of response for all physicians in the community. If the approach became popular, it would be necessary to organize additional experts from the practicing community who would act as educational consultants with help from medical school faculty members.

Role in Patient Education

It is likely that medical schools will have significant involvement with patient or public education. The details of this will be left to other chapters.

Nonphysician Health Professionals

Concepts such as the Community Hospital Network can serve health professionals in addition to physicians. Nurses and clinical pharmacists could be particularly well served. The chief role of medical schools in this regard will be in teaching and training the practicing physician to better instruct other members of the health care team.

Certifying and Licensing Bodies

The trend toward recertification and relicensure is continuing. Attendance in approved courses of continuing education and paper-and-pencil tests are two popular methods for meeting these new requirements. Medical schools can offer a service to the profession and their patients by experimenting with other approaches. For example, physicians practicing in hospitals with meaningful education based on audit and evaluation feedback might be recertified and relicensed on this basis. As methodologies in problem identification become refined, the medical office will become a center of continuing education. It is possible that participation in this type of practice will prove more meaningful in the assurance of excellent patient care than a certifying examination or attendance at a course. The proposed medical school research and development centers would need to organize trials to determine the best methods available.

Summary

The position is taken that medical schools should have a formalized central position in CME. Research and development of techniques of determining educational needs through automatic and noninvasive quality assurance linked with practice-based continuing education will be a major role for medical schools. Research and development centers should be developed in eight or ten medical schools to help determine the most effective and efficient methods. This approach is essential if future legislation involving continuing education is to be based on sound principles. Emphasis should be on the development of the concept of a true continuum of education with faculty, resident, and medical student practice being organized into models which allow identification of need and appropriate educational and organizational responses to these needs. Medical schools can also form networks with community hospitals that desire to become intramural teaching centers. It is probable that with proper organization and financial support these activities can be carried out by medical schools without an unrealistic drain on faculty time.

ROLE OF THE MEDICAL SOCIETIES

Medical societies can play an important role in facilitating meaningful CME. Medical societies can, in general, support continuing medical education that is linked to quality assurance. They can define proper standards of practice while guarding against harsh punitive treatment of the profession so that continuing medical education and quality assurance can continue to be used to improve patient care rather than become a destructive force or a wasteful bureaucratic circus. Generally, medical societies have begun to get significantly involved in continuing education and in most situations appear to be moving more rapidly than medical schools.

American Medical Association

The American Medical Association continues to be in a key position. The AMA can effectively support continuing medical education by encouraging physicians to participate in meaningful quality assurance programs. The AMA can serve as a coordinating device for general standards of health care and can, in particular, coordinate standards for those physicians who do not participate in one of the specialty organizations.

State and Local Societies

State and local societies are appropriate bodies to coordinate continuing medical education and quality assurance activities within their states. In large states they can help coordinate the efforts of the medical schools. They can encourage studies which determine true needs of the profession and can further refine standards from the state level. A farsighted state society, such as the California Medical Association, can provide useful service to its members by staying active in CME and facilitating proper research by the medical schools and, in some cases, the association itself.

Specialty Societies

Specialty societies such as the American College of Physicians, American Heart Association, American College of Cardiology, American College of Surgeons, American Academy of Family Practice and many others are best suited to outline standards for their specialty. They are able to help organize, with the National Board of Medical Examiners, self-assessment examinations of cognitive knowledge and determine specific recertification requirements. These societies, working closely with medical faculty, can effectively develop and encourage the development of the organization of specialty practice so it most efficiently takes its place in the big picture of health care delivery in the United States. The specialty societies appear to be reacting favorably to the new challenges of continuing education.

The Association of American Medical Colleges

The interinstitutional organization, the Association of American Medical Colleges (AAMC), must play a very significant role if continuing education is to develop its useful potential. The AAMC can help define and formulate the roles of medical schools in continuing education and can, of course, coordinate activities among medical schools. It also provides a forum in which medical school faculty interested in continuing medical education can develop their own continuing education based on defined needs and solutions to these problems. The AAMC must become a powerful spokesman for continuing education on behalf of medical schools.

ROLE OF HOSPITALS

Quality assurance and utilization review within hospitals have paved the way for more useful activities which will emphasize improvement of patient care rather than merely cost containment. It is probable that the community hospital is the best site for most continuing medical education. The most important contribution for the community hospital in continuing education is through assessment of hospital records and patient outcomes. It is therefore important that hospitals insist that records be auditable and that educational experiences or organizational changes be undertaken when specific needs are identified. The hospital should be the grass roots for evolution and implementation of standards.

For its CME program it would be best if each community hospital could be linked with a medical school. The medical school could serve as a stimulus and resource to help the community hospital develop into an intramural teaching center.

The future of PSROs is discussed in other chapters. This program might be most useful in stimulating education in hospital practice, although it currently appears to be more involved with cost containment.

ROLE OF THE COMPUTER

The conflict over the tendency to continue traditional forms of postgraduate programs as opposed to emphasis on determination of educational needs and problem solving can be reduced by existing computer technology. The proper use of computers can greatly diminish the need for transmitting information when it is not needed or will not be used. Existing computer systems can provide information to the physician at the time he needs it for problem solving, while he is actually developing his plans for diagnosis and therapy. This computer display of information at the time of problem solving is surely more valuable than the memory based approach of teaching facts in a postgraduate course several months before they are needed, or after the fact from retrospective audit.

The proper utilization of the computer as a tool thus promises a breakthrough which will minimize the need to base continuing education on transmission of information in courses or by audio-visual devices.

Medical schools, medical societies, and hospitals should stimulate further experimental and developmental models that will facilitate the use of the computer as a tool for the physician in problem solving. The experience of Dr. Lawrence Weed[17],[18] in the experimental use of the computer on the obstetrical service at the University of Vermont should be extended and brought to the community hospital and possibly the physician's office for further testing, development, and refinement. If there is conflict about the most useful computer system, several models should be tested.

Role for Future Planning and Monitoring

No system of education should exist without a mechanism for monitoring progress and planning for progress. Numerous organizations desire and will need a role in monitoring and planning the new look in continuing education. The AAMC will be a strong force in this area. Each state should form a coordination committee, federation, or organization composed of members from different societies and organizations such as the LCCME. This committee can monitor CME activities and plan for future growth at the state level while relating to the LCCME nationwide. On the national scene, the LCCME is in the most advantageous position to coordinate monitoring and planning.

NOTES

1. George E. Miller, "Continuing Education for What?" *Journal of Medical Education* 42 (April 1967): 320-326.

2. John W. Williamson, Marshall Alexander, and George E. Miller, "Continuing Education and Patient Care Research," *JAMA* 201 (September 18, 1967): 118-122.

3. John W. Williamson, Marshall Alexander, and George E. Miller, "Priorities in Patient-Care Research and Continuing Medical Education," *JAMA* 204 (April 22, 1968): 93-98.

4. John W. Williamson, "Evaluating Quality of Patient Care," *JAMA* 218 (October 25, 1971): 564-569.

5. Joseph S. Gonnella *et al.*, "Evaluation of Patient Care," *JAMA* 214 (December 14, 1970): 2040-2043.

6. C.R. Brown, Jr., and D.S. Fleisher, "The Bi-Cycle Concept— Relating Continuing Education Directly to Patient Care," *New England Journal of Medicine* (May 20, 1971): 88-97.

7. O.L. Peterson *et al.*, "An Analytical Study of North Carolina General Practice, 1953-54," *JAMA* 31, Part II (1956): 1-165.

8. Modified from Report, "4th Annual California Medical Association Planning and Goals Conference," San Diego, California, November 1975.

9. Malcolm S. Knowles, *The Modern Practice of Adult Education: Andragogy Versus Pedagogy* (New York: The Association Press, 1970), p. 38.

10. Phil R. Manning, Stephen Abrahamson, and Donald A. Dennis, "Research in Medical Education—Comparison of Four Teaching Techniques: Programmed Text, Textbook, Lecture-Demonstration, and Lecture Workshop," *Journal of Medical Education* 43 (March 1968): 356-359.

11. Phil R. Manning, "Pre and Post Course Testing as a Teaching Aid," *The Mayo Alumnus* 2 (January 1966): 18-20.

12. Charles E. Lewis and Ruth S. Hassanein, "Continuing Medical Education—An Epidemiologic Evaluation," *New England Journal of Medicine* 282 (1970): 254-259.

13. Thomas Meyer, *A Feasibility Study in Determining Individual Practice Profiles of Physicians as a Basis for Continuing Education of These Physicians Utilizing a Postgraduate Preceptor Technique,* A Final Report (Madison, Wisconsin: University of Wisconsin, 1970), p.32.

14. Sigurd E. Sivertson *et al.*, "Individual Physician Profile: Continuing Education Related to Medical Practice," *Journal of Medical Education* 48, (November 1973): 1006-1012.

15. D. Hamaty, "West Virginia State Medical Association's Voluntary Peer Review Service," *West Virginia Medical Journal* 66 (September 1970): 307-309, 323-329.

16. Warren Williams, personal communication at the meeting of Medical College's Directors of Continuing Education, April 1, 1976, La Costa, California.

17. Lawrence L. Weed, "Conference on Trends and Medical Education," Report, Macy Foundation Conference, Colorado, September 1975.

18. Stephen V. Cantrill, "A Problem-oriented Medical Information System," in *The Problem Oriented System* (New York: Medcom, Inc., 1972) pp. 268-273.

Chapter 18
Patient Education, Patient Compliance and the Continuing Education of Physicians

Philip R. Lee

The relationship of continuing medical education to the quality of patient care is unclear.[1] Even though there is little direct evidence of any positive correlation between continuing medical and clinical competence, a growing number of state medical societies and other professional associations are stressing its importance. A few, such as those in Oregon and Arizona, require their members to attend CME programs as a condition of continued membership, and the Board of Family Practice requires CME for recertification. Following the lead of the medical profession, a number of states now require participation in continuing education programs for relicensure.

A new approach is needed, one that includes many of the elements of present models but is based on patients' needs rather than physicians' needs. An approach based on a cooperative educational program, including patient, pharmacist, and physician participation and the use of patient package inserts is proposed as an alternative to present models of CME. Patient package inserts would be used to facilitate patient education and drug counseling by pharmacists and physicians. The program should be evaluated in relation to the patient's, the pharmacist's, and the physician's knowledge about the disease to be treated, the drugs to be used, and their possible adverse effects. It should also be evaluated in terms of patient compliance with the prescribed regimen, control of the disease, and adverse drug reactions.

Existing problems that a drug-specific patient education program would aim to correct include: inadequate physician and patient knowledge about drugs, irrational prescribing, adverse drug reactions, and poor patient compliance with prescribed regimens. These problems are deeply rooted in medical education and in the influence of the pharmaceutical industry on the continuing education of physicians, as well as on patient behavior.

HOW ARE PHYSICIANS INFORMED ABOUT DRUGS?

Physicians attempt to maintain their clinical competence in the use of prescription drugs through a variety of means. A sound medical education is the foundation for this process. There is little doubt that medical education in the United States, at its best, is unequalled anywhere. Yet, there is a healthy climate of criticism that recognizes that this training is not always adequate, and a variety of new approaches are being undertaken to determine how to improve medical education. Improvements are surely needed in the teaching of pharmacology and in clinical pharmacology. Only a handful of medical schools maintain outstanding training programs in clinical pharmacology.

Perhaps even more important than the urgent need to improve drug educational programs in the medical schools is the need to improve clinical pharmacology training for interns, residents, and practicing physicians. Too often in teaching hospitals the most readily available source of prescription information is the *Physicians' Desk Reference*, rather than the hospital formulary or a text on clinical pharmacology. Drug detailmen are a frequent source of information for physicians in training. Well-trained clinical pharmacists could provide more objective information related to the care of individual patients.

Interns and residents, like practicing physicians, obtain information on prescription drugs from many sources: medical journals; journals of prescribing, such as *The Medical Letter* and *Pharmacology for Physicians* or the *FDA Drug Bulletin;* drug compendia, such as the *Physicians' Desk Reference* and the *Merck Manual;* formularies; textbooks; industry advertising; the material accompanying drug samples; the presentations of detailmen; postgraduate education; and consultation with colleagues. The drug-industry-supported detailmen and the *Physicians' Desk Reference*, a book consisting of paid advertising material, are the sources most often used for prescribing information. Industry supported journals, seminars, exhibits, and educational materials add to the dominant influence of the pharmaceutical industry.

Recently, the role of the pharmaceutical industry was reviewed by Crout, who described the extent of industry support of journals distributed without charge to physicians, the content of many of these journals promoting the use of drugs, as well as industry's support of seminars and scientific meetings and the development of educational materials for physicians. In analyzing these developments he observed:

> The proliferation of industry-supported educational material
> has increased to the point where they now constitute the bulk
> of educational material provided to the practicing physician
> in his practice.[2]

The role of the pharmaceutical industry is evident in the magnitude of its promotional efforts directed toward physicians. It has been estimated by Rucker that drug promotion expenditures exceed $1.3 billion annually, including over $790 million to support the activities of drug detailmen.[3] (Whether this can be legitimately related to the continuing education of physicians, it does influence prescribing habits.)

Crout decried the influence of commercial interests on the postgraduate education of the medical profession. As others before him who have examined the issues, he found no easy solutions "without major changes in the whole structure of post-graduate medical education."[4]

Although physicians have a great deal of information available about prescription drugs, and many use it well and prescribe rationally, the prescribing habits of too many physicians result too often in the misuse of prescription drugs, poor patient compliance with prescribed regimens, and adverse drug reactions. Also, despite the wealth of available information, physician knowledge of frequently prescribed drugs is much less than it should be. In a recent test of physician knowledge of antibiotics, only 11 percent of physicians in practice over 15 years or more scored 80 percent or higher, thereby equalling the average score of university-affiliated doctors.[5]

One dimension of the situation results from an excess of information and insufficient time to carefully evaluate it. This torrent of drug information is, at least in part, a reflection of the explosion in scientific knowledge and technology that has occurred in the last forty years, providing an unprecedented number and variety of new drug products.

Various programs to improve medical education and the availability of objective information about drugs for practicing physicians have been proposed,[6] but they have not proved sufficient to deal with the

198 QUALITY HEALTH CARE

problems related to the irrational prescribing and misuse of prescription drugs. Recently, Rucker proposed the establishment of a National Drug Information Foundation to provide drug information to physicians and pharmacists. A basic element in the proposed program would be 2,000 therapeutic consultants to supply practitioners with objective, comparative information about drugs that are relevant for their type of practice.[7] A more realistic scheme than that of the therapeutic consultants suggested by Rucker would be one involving community pharmacists who could play a far more active role in drug education services for physicians and patients.

IRRATIONAL PRESCRIBING

Since the hearings held in the late 1960s by the late Senator Estes Kefauver, Senator Gaylord Nelson, and their colleagues and the publication of the reports of the HEW Task Force on Prescription Drugs in 1968 and 1969, it has become increasingly apparent that much prescribing has been and is irrational. Antibiotics and other antimicrobial agents — some costly and all carrying a risk to the patient — have been prescribed prophylactically without evidence of potential value. They have been prescribed for the common cold and other minor upper respiratory infections; they have been prescribed over the telephone to patients not examined by the physicians; they have been prescribed without appropriate cultures; and they have been prescribed for a variety of conditions for which they are clinically worthless. All in all, antibiotics and other anti-infectives account for from 15 to 20 percent of all new and refill prescriptions in community pharmacies.

In hospitals, 20 to 40 percent of all patients receive an antibiotic during their hospital stay. Many patients (30 to 60 percent in some studies) on surgical wards receive antibiotics prophylactically or without clear-cut indications. By any standards, these numbers appear excessive. Tetracyclines continue to be prescribed extensively for children below the age of eight years without adequate indication, despite the fact that adverse effects of tetracycline therapy have been known for years and despite the warning that has been included in the package insert since 1970. In 1973, enough tetracycline was certified to treat 2.6 million children with one gram per day for five days. Following a study of the problem, the Committee on Drugs of the American Academy of Pediatrics concluded: "There are few if any reasons for using tetracycline drugs in children less than eight years old."[8] Even more alarming is the continued, widespread prescribing of chloramphenicol. Although much less widely used than in years past, many physicians continue to prescribe it, rarely with adequate or appropriate indications.

Numerous other drugs have been used for many years, often with high endorsements by both physicians and patients, even though later studies demonstrated that the products were only "possibly effective" or were "ineffective." Effective but dangerous drugs are prescribed when equally effective but safer agents are available. Two drugs, each known to be safe when used alone have been given in combination to the same patient, causing a serious or fatal (drug-drug) interaction. Drugs are offered for the same patient by one physician or by several different physicians in excessive quantities. Patients with known drug allergies are given the drugs to which they are allergic. Patients are given prescriptions when, on rational grounds, no prescription of any kind is needed. Other patients are given no prescriptions, or inadequate regimens are prescribed when effective drugs are available (e.g., hypertension).

ADVERSE DRUG REACTIONS

These irrational prescribing habits have been implicated in serious adverse drug reactions that can require hospitalization; extend the hospital stay of a patient; cause pain, tissue damage, temporary or permanent disability, and even death.

Estimates of the morbidity, mortality, and cost of adverse drug reactions vary widely. Part of the problem relates to the definitions used and part to the methods applied and the patients studied. Melmon and Morelli use the term "drug reaction" to mean "all unwanted consequences of drug administration, even administration of the wrong drug (or drugs), to the wrong patient in the wrong dosage (form, amount, route or interval), at the wrong time, or for the wrong disease."[9] Few have adopted this definition. In many respects, this definition is the antithesis of the HEW Prescription Drug Task Force's definition of rational prescribing.[10] It goes well beyond currently accepted definitions of adverse drug reactions. If this definition were used, the magnitude of the problem would be far larger than is reflected in most current studies of adverse drug reactions.

The most widely accepted definition of adverse drug reaction is "any response to a drug which is noxious and unintended and which occurs at doses used in man for prophylaxis, diagnosis or therapy, excluding therapeutic failures."[11]

In examining the literature on adverse drug reactions, Karsh and Lasagna felt it was not possible to extrapolate the available data from limited hospital or outpatient clinic studies to provide valid estimates of the adverse drug reaction problem in the United States.[12] They examined data on adverse drug reactions in hospitalized patients, hospital admissions due to adverse drug reactions, and fatal drug reactions. Although it is not possible to extrapolate data from a number of hospital or outpatient studies to the population of the United States, there is ample evidence to indicate that adverse drug reactions are a serious problem and are a direct or contributing cause of considerable morbidity and mortality. Much of this is preventable.

PATIENT ATTITUDES AND ACTIONS— THE PROBLEM OF COMPLIANCE

Patients cannot escape the charge that they, by their actions and attitudes, have contributed to the problems of drug misuse, adverse drug reactions, and poor compliance. Part of this can be attributed to the patients' demand for drugs, and part to the alarmingly high rate of error among patients in the self-administration of prescription drugs.

A large number of studies have been published describing the problems of patient noncompliance with a variety of medical regimens.[13,14] Noncompliance could be manifest in failure to keep appointments, failure to take medications as prescribed, or failure to follow the total regimen proposed by the physician. Patients with symptomatic disease are more likely to keep appointments and follow prescribed regimens than patients with asymptomatic disease (e.g., hypertension).

Most studies have shown that about 20 percent of patients with symptomatic disease fail to keep appointments as compared with as many as 50 percent of patients with asymptomatic disease. A wide range of noncompliance with prescribed regimens has been found. Most studies show that 25 to 50 percent of patients do not comply with prescribed regimens; some show a figure as low as 15 percent.

In a study reported from the University of Florida, more than 20 percent of diabetic patients were taking either one-half or double the prescribed dose of insulin. Almost 50 percent of the patients with tuberculosis admitted taking their medication irregularly or not at all, and in a group told to take antibiotics regularly to control a streptococal infection 56 percent decided on their own to stop therapy by the third day, 71 percent by the sixth day, and 82 percent by the ninth day.[15] In a study of patients with congestive heart failure reported by

Marsh and Perlman,[16] it was found that only slightly over half of the patients took their digitalis as prescribed. The results of a number of studies of compliance by diabetes mellitus patients regarding recommended measures as to diet, medication, urine testing, and foot care revealed that "...overall, less than 10 percent of the patients observed were carrying out a minimally adequate regimen in all of theses areas of day-to-day management of their diabetes."[17] The most common failures in patient compliance appear to be omission of doses or the premature discontinuance of therapy.

A summary of the magnitude of patient compliance with therapeutic regimens indicates a mean of about 50 percent with a wide variance.[18] Apparently about one-third of the patients always comply, about one-third never comply, and about one-third comply sometimes. A variety of patient behaviors are included in noncompliance:

- They are told to take three tablets a day, but decide to take fifteen, perhaps on the grounds that if three is good, fifteen must be five times better.
- They forget to take their medicine for a week and then take a week's supply at once.
- They are instructed to take the drug before meals, but they take it after meals. (Even when they are anxious to follow instructions, they may not be sure whether "before meals" means fifteen minutes before, one hour before, or three hours before.)
- They are warned not to use a drug for more than a week, but they take it for three weeks to "give it a little more time to have an effect."
- They have combined antihistamine cold remedies, nose drops, or sedatives with presumably moderate quantities of alcohol or a barbiturate and killed not only themselves, but other victims in automobile collisions.
- They forget to tell their physician about other prescription or nonprescription drugs they might be taking.
- They fail to report to their physician the first apparent symptoms of what may be an adverse reaction.
- They treat themselves with a drug prescribed for someone else in the family or a friendly neighbor.

Although patient education is a factor in noncompliance[19] and patients share much of the blame, they cannot be given full responsibility. Too often, physicians have neglected to explain what a prescribed drug is supposed to do, how it should be taken, and what the most important side effects may be. Too often, physicians are unaware that a patient is so apprehensive during a visit that he or she will promptly forget whatever warnings were given. Too often, physicians are unaware that a prescription labeled simply "take as directed" can become totally meaningless after a few weeks or months have passed.

Pharmacists have an excellent opportunity to discuss prescriptions with patients — supporting and amplifying the physician's instructions, intensifying the warnings, explaining how the particular product should be stored, describing the importance of the expiration date on the package. They can do this in simple terminology and in a setting that causes little or no apprehension. Unfortunately, however, they seldom take advantage of this opportunity.

The problems of patient noncompliance with prescribed regimens are often not recognized by the physician.[20] When they are recognized, they are usually blamed on poor patient cooperation, lack of patient motivation, or patient ignorance. The physician often overlooks his or her own role in the matter.

In a study of the role of mass media and patient counseling by a group at Stanford University, a number of factors were found to be of importance in achieving informed patient cooperation. These include: awareness, motivation, information, instruction, and reinforcement.[21] Patient understanding is a critical factor. B. Blackwell observed: "The most important contribution to compliance is the understanding a patient has of the illness, the need for treatment and the likely consequences of both."[22]

To provide the patient with this information the physician must be a teacher, and to do an effective job of teaching, the physician must be actively studying. A variety of approaches to improving patient compliance, including patient education, have been proposed. The role of the physician, the patient, and the medical regimen have been stressed by D. Mathews[23] and L. Lasagna.[24] The modalities of patient education, personality accommodation, family involvement, group methods, and regimen negotiation are stressed by R. F. Gillum and A. J. Barsky.[25] R. N. Podell emphasized that the failure of the physician to pursue aggressive therapy despite a poorly controlled blood pressure was a major factor in patient noncompliance.[26]

Most patient education is done in the physician's office. In addition to the physician, a nurse, dietician, physician therapist, or other health professional can be involved. The physician usually has limited time to instruct the patient and can seldom provide in-depth information or adequate follow-up.

Organized classes and courses are sometimes provided, usually by large group practices, hospitals, or physicians dealing with patients with special problems. Obstetricians have long conducted group sessions for pregnant women on subjects ranging from diet and exercise to nursing the infant. Other organized classes are usually for diabetics, cardiacs, or other patients with serious disease or disability. A few state and local health departments are active in the field of patient education. Voluntary associations, such as the American Diabetes Association, the American Cancer Society, and the American Heart Association have been active both in general consumer health education and in the development of materials that can be used for patient education.

Informed consent decisions by the courts have resulted in an increasing effort on the part of the physician to instruct and inform patients prior to surgery. The need in other areas of therapy, particularly the use of prescription drugs, has not been stressed.

As might be expected, drug companies have also developed educational materials that can be used for both group and individual instruction. Some of the more innovative of these approaches to patient education include:

- the "Activated Patient" program developed by K. W. Shenert at Georgetown University Medical School;[27]
- behavior modification programs for obese patients as pioneered by A. J. Stunkard;[28]
- the use of nurse practitioners in the treatment of hypertensive patients as pioneered by F. A. Finnerty;[29] and
- the professional/patient contract developed by a group of diabetes specialists as a stimulus and guide to active patient participation.[30]

The development of disease-specific, clinically tested teaching and evaluation protocols will be essential for future third party reimbursement, accreditation by the Joint Commission on Accreditation of Hospitals, and/or evaluation by Professional Standards Review Organizations.[31]

A program of physician and pharmacist continuing education focusing on rational prescribing and patient compliance, using the patient package insert as an important element in the program, might help to reduce irrational prescribing, patient noncompliance, and adverse drug reactions. The program should be disease- or drug-specific; and it should include the following objectives: increased patient awareness, motivation, information, instruction, and reinforcement; improved physician and pharmacist knowledge of the disease and drugs used to treat it; improved prescribing and dispensing; and improved disease control with fewer adverse drug reactions.

The problem of meeting the need is enormous. It is estimated that about 70 million individuals regularly use prescription or over-the-counter drugs. The average number of prescriptions per person per year has risen from 2.4 in 1950 to 6.6 in 1974. Among the millions of adults who take drugs regularly there are 15 million who use aspirin, 10 million who use antihypertensive drugs, and 5 million who use oral contraceptives. Other drugs taken regularly by large numbers of adults include diazapam, antacids, digoxin, prednisone, and warfarin. In the development of patient education programs and patient package inserts, priority should be given to those classes of drugs, such as antihypertensives, analgesics, psychoactive drugs, antibiotics, digitalis preparations, steroids, anticoagulants, and antacids that are widely used.

THE ROLE OF THE PHYSICIAN AND THE PHARMACIST IN PATIENT EDUCATION

Too little attention has been paid to the potential of physician-pharmacist cooperation in patient education. A number of studies have demonstrated improved patient compliance with therapeutic regimens when the patients have been given specific written instructions or have been involved in disease-specific health education programs.[32]

The use of pharmacists in counseling patients on the use of drugs is increasing rapidly, but it is still the exception rather than the rule. Patients do not ordinarily view their own pharmacist as a source of information about prescription drugs, yet the pharmacist's assistance can be just as vital as the physician's in achieving the desired results of therapy. One recently reported study, for example, showed that 29 percent of patients not given drug counseling failed to comply with instructions, as compared with 3.4 percent of counseled patients. In another group of patients, 20.8 percent of a control group had an error rate in the use of antimicrobial drugs in excess of 50 percent but only 5.8 percent of patients counseled by pharmacists had a comparable error rate.[33] The pharmacist-counselor's impact is based on the ability to improve patient understanding of the medication regimen. A patient who does not have at least a rudimentary knowledge of his or her regimen is fare more likely to commit errors in the use of pre-scribeddrugs. In addition to patient instruction, special packaging of medications has also been found to be useful in achieving increased patient compliance with therapeutic regimens.[34]

A number of recent studies have demonstrated the importance of patient education in achieving compliance with antihypertensives regimens. In one group of patients counseled by a pharmacist, the proportion of patients taking at least 90 percent of their prescribed medication increased from 25 to 79 percent, and the percentage of patients who were normotensive increased from 20 to 79 percent. The controls showed either no change or a decrease in control of blood pressure. Although the gains were not maintained after the active counseling of the patients was discontinued, the patients who were in the counseled group had an average blood pressure significantly below that of the control group.[35] In commenting on the role of the pharmacist in counseling these patients, R.N. Podell and L.R. Gary noted:

> ... one, or more, of the continuous activities of the pharmacist was critical: clarifying instructions, monitoring compliance, eliciting negative feedback, adjusting the medical regimen, and focusing the physician's attention on compliance and blood pressure control. Curiously enough, each activity done by the pharmacist in this case could and should also be performed by the physician. One lesson is that either the physician or a physician substitute needs to serve in an effective compliance role.[36]

The only thing that might have been added to further involve the patient would be the patient's measurement of blood pressure at home and dosage adjustment after consultation with physician or pharmacist. Certainly the primary care physician could have carried out the same program of patient instruction, but too few of them do this at the present time.

The problem for the physician was presented clearly by S.C. Sheps and R.A. Kirkpatrick:

> More refined vasodilator drugs and new agents such as the prostaglandins and angiotensin antagonists are being developed, and more and more people are learning about hypertension. But unprescribed drugs or disregarded prescriptions do not control hypertension, and people forget what they learn—so the key to controlling hypertension may

> be the interest and motivation of the physician himself. Without his vital concern and thoughtful flexibility in individualizing treatment, no therapeutic regimen or public education program can remain effective.[37]

The importance of the physician's attitude and behavior in achieving patient compliance in the treatment of hypertension has also been stressed bx T.S. Inui, E.L. Yourtee, and J.W. Williamson.[38] The objectives are to provide the patient with the information needed to take responsibility for his or her health and the management of his or her illness, to improve compliance with the prescribed regimens, to reduce irrational prescribing and drug misuse, to improve control of the disease, and to reduce adverse drug reactions.

In the efforts to cope with these complex problems, the pharmicist and the physician both have important roles to play. The physician must first make the diagnosis or define the problems and determine the appropriate therapy. The physician should inform the patient about the diagnosis, the treatment plan, and the medication prescribed. The pharmacist should supplement the information and counseling provided by the physician. The pharmacist should be given the responsibility for giving the patient package insert to the patient and for counseling the patient about the drugs prescribed. Problems of compliance and drug reactions should be discussed. Usually, the pharmacist has more time than does the physician to discuss the material with the patient. In many, and perhaps most, cases, it is the pharmacist who is more knowledgeable about how each drug should be taken and stored, as well as about potential interactions with other drugs. It is also the pharmacist who might be aware of other physicians the patient is consulting, and which other drug product (prescription or over the counter) the patient might be using. In either case, merely providing the patient with the written patient package insert or with information about drugs verbally will have little effect on patient compliance. Continuing education of the patient with periodic reinforcement is the key.

In providing written material for patients, particularly patient package inserts, every step should be taken to prevent needless patient alarm or confusion. Certainly, the long detailed information presented to physicians and pharmacists in the present package inserts would be inappropriate. Consideration should be given to the decision of whether to include all indications approved by FDA for each drug, or only the most important or most frequent indications. There would appear to be no justification for listing all the warnings, contraindications, and potential adverse reactions, known or suspected. Presenting this torrent of information to patients would be a serious disservice. Careful study should be given to the desirability of including only the most serious side effects, or the most frequent, or some combination of these.

In some instances, the physician could be dealing with patients who would be placed under emotional stress if they read about possible adverse effects of the drugs they should take. This problem can be dealt with if the physician specifies in writing on the prescription that a particular patient should not be given the patient package insert with instructions by the pharmacist.

The patient package insert would not only provide an additional source of drug information for the physician and the patient but its availability would help stimulate greater cooperation among physician, patient, and pharmacist in the prescribing, dispensing, and use of prescription drugs. To be successful, this educational effort will have to involve physician, pharmacist, and patient as active participants. Simply delivering written information to the patient, by either pharmacist or physician, will not produce the desired patient compliance or reduce adverse drug reactions. Instructions should be reviewed in writing until the patient demonstrates an understanding of the instructions. In cases of chronic illness, periodic review or reassessment is essential. Written instructions cannot replace physician-patient and pharmacist-patient interactions, but they should be an integral part of the transaction.

This approach to patient, pharmacist, and physician education must be part of a broader strategy to deal with the many complex social, economic, political, and medical problems related to the use of prescription and over-the-counter drugs.[39] The approach suggested has an advantage over many other programs of continuing education and quality assurance in that it can be evaluated objectively. It has the additional advantage that it might help relate programs of drug education to patient needs and not merely the needs of physician, pharmacist, or pharmaceutical industry.

NOTES

1. Richard Greene, *Assuring Quality in Medical Care: The State of the Art* (Cambridge, Mass.: Ballinger Publishing Co., 1976), p. 293.

2. S.R. Crout, Testimony before Monopoly Subcommittee, Small Business Committee, U.S. Senate, April 26, 1976, p. 39.

3. T.D. Rucker, "Drug Information for Prescribers and Dispensers," *Medical Care* 14 (February 1976): 165.

4. Crout, *op. cit.*, p. 37.

5. H.C. Neu and S.P. Howrey "Testing the Physician's Knowledge of Antibiotic Use: Self-Assessment and Learning Via Videotape," *New England Journal of Medicine* 293 (December 18, 1975): 1293-1295.

6. HEW Task Force on Prescription Drugs, *Final Report* (Washington, D.C.: Department of Health, Education and Welfare, 1969), p. 86.

7. Rucker, *op. cit.*, pp. 156-165.

8. S.J. Yaffe *et al*, "Requiem for Tetracyclines," *Pediatrics* 55 (1975): 142-143.

9. K. Melmon and H. Morrelli, *Clinical Pharmacology: Basic Principles in Therapeutics* (New York: The Macmillan Co., 1972), p. 570.

10. Task Force on Prescription Drugs; *op. cit.*, p. 21.

11. F. Karsh and L. Lasagna, *Adverse Drug Reactions in the United States* (Washington, D.C.: Medicine in Public Interest, 1974), p. 2.

12. *Ibid.*, p. 28.

13. R.B. Haynes and D.L. Saucett, *An Annotated Bibliography on the Compliance of Patients with Therapeutic Regimens* (Hamilton, Ontario: McMaster University Medical School, 1974).

14. R.M Podell, *Physician's Guide to Compliance in Hypertension* (West Point, Pennsylvania: Merck and Company, Inc., 1975), p. 97.

15. R.B. Stewart and L.E. Cluff, "A Review of Medication Errors and Compliance in Ambulant Patients," *Clinical Pharmacology and Therapeutics* 13 (July-August 1972): 463.

16. W.W. Marsh and L.V. Perlman, "Understanding Congestive Heart Failure and Self Administration of Digoxin," Abstracted in A.I. Wertheimer and M.C. Smith, *Pharmacy Practice: Social and Behavioral Aspects* (Baltimore, Md.: University Park Press, 1974), p. 202.

17. T.F. Williams, "Needs for Diabetes Education," in G. Steiner and P. Lawrence, *Handbook on the Education of the Diabetic Patient* (to be published).

18. D.L. Sackett, *A Workshop Symposium: Compliance with Therapeutic Regimens* (Hamilton, Ontario: McMaster University Medical Center, May 1974), p. 3.

19. Marsh and Perlman, *op. cit.*, pp. 202-203.

20. M. Weintraub, W.Y.N. Au, and L. Lasagna, "Compliance as a Determinant of Serum Digoxin Concentration," *JAMA* 224 (April 1973): 481-485.

21. J.W. Farquhar, personal communication.

22. B. Blackwell, "Patient Compliance," *New England Journal of Medicine* 289 (August 2, 1973): 249-252.

23. Daryl Matthews, "The Noncompliant Patient,"*Primary Care* 2 (August 2, 1973): 289-294.

24. Louis Lasagna, "Fault and Default'," *New England Journal of Medicine* 289 (August 2, 1973): 267-268.

25. R.F. Gillum and A.J. Barsky, "Diagnosis and Management of Patient Noncompliance," *JAMA* 228 (June 17, 1974): 1563-1567.

26. Podell, *op. cit.*, p. 46.

27. K.W. Shenert and H. Eisenberg, *How to Be Your Own Doctor—Sometimes* (New York: Crosset and Dunlap, 1975), p. 353.

28. A.J. Stunkard, *The Pain of Obesity* (Palo Alto: Bull Publishing Company, 1976), p. 236.

29. F.A. Finnerty, "The Nurse and The Care of the Hypertensive Patient," *Annals of Internal Medicine* 84 (June 1976): 746.

30. D.D Etzwiler, ed., *Education and Management of the Patient with Diabetes Mellitus* (Elkhart, Indiana: Ames Co., 1973).

31. Task Force on Consumer Health Education, *Toward a National Policy of Health Promotion and Consumer Health Education* (Washington, D.C.; Fogarty International Center, National Institutes of Health, June 1975), Chapter Two, p. 11 (to be published).

32. R. Greene, J. Simmons, and J. Golden, "The Role of Consumer Behavior in the Outcome of Health Services Interventions," in R. Greene, *Assuring Quality in Medical Care: The State of the Art* (Cambridge, Mass.: Ballinger Publishing Co., 1976), pp. 257-270.

33. E.E. Madden, "Evaluation of Outpatient Pharmacy Patient Counseling," *Journal of the American Pharmaceutical Association* 13 (August 1973): 437-443.

34. R.B. Catalano and H.L. Flack, "Effect of Packaging and and Instruction on Outpatient Compliance with Medication Regimens," *Drug Intell. Clin. Pharm.* 8 (January 1974): 10-15.

35. J.M. McKenney *et al.*, "The Effect of Clinical Pharmacy Services on Patients with Essential Hypertension," *Circulation* 48 (1973): 1104-1111.

36. R.N. Podell and L.R. Gary, "Hypertension and Compliance Implica-

tions for the Primary Physician," *New England Journal of Medicine* 294 (May 13, 1976): 1120-1121.

37. Sheps and Kirkpatrick, *op. cit.*, p. 719.

38. T.S. Inui, E.L. Yourtee, and J.W. Williamson, "Improved Outcomes in Hypertension after Physician Tutorials," *Annals of Internal Medicine* 84 (June 1976): 646-651.

39. M. Silverman and P.R. Lee, *Pills, Profits and Politics* (Berkeley: University of California Press, 1974), p. 403.

Chapter 19
Health Education for Consumers: An Alternative to Continuing Education for Providers

Rick J. Carlson

The subject matter of this book is continuing medical education—of professionals, not patients. Yet, in their perverse desire for "diversity of opinion," the editors have asked me to address a different question. They have asked that I consider whether "continuing education of the public" is an alternative to continuing education of the provider. This could prove to be a mistake; it is a sleeping giant of a question. Indeed, we must be very clear about what this question really means.

The beginning of the end of the classical Roman church was the sale of indulgences. As the church lurched its way into Sybaritism and excess, it got caught in a cash flow crunch. New monies were needed to feed its growth and appetites. What better idea than to "bicen-tennialize" the means of salvation; but how profoundly coun-terintuitive! The sale of indulgences was a signal to the lowly parishioner that the church could be bought—no longer was the road to heaven paved with unswerving faith and gobs of good deeds. Just the purchase of a few icons and trinkets was every bit as good. But what a tawdry salvation that was. No longer was the church in all its magnificent trappings the arbiter of the soul's passage. Now the in-dividual could do something about it.

This loss of "mystique" was not just an idle historical moment; it led to the Reformation. It only took someone as compulsive as Martin Luther to figure out that the Church had gone out on a limb—he cut it off by simply pointing out that redemption was a matter of faith, not conspicuous consumption. The Church never quite recovered.

The same sort of danger is present here.[1] Can anyone take seriously the idea that instead of trying to sharpen the skills of providers to minister to ignorant consumers, the attempt should rather be made to teach consumers to become less ignorant? This is a patent heresy and must be recognized as such.

Yet I am afraid I am stuck with the task. The editors have assigned me this responsibility, perhaps unaware of the grave dangers. Reluctantly then, this chapter explores the possibility of consumer education — if not as an alternative to professional education, at least as a complementary tool. May the Martin Luthers of our time be caught napping!

THE EVIDENCE

To repeat, the task is to examine the relative benefits of continuing education of professionals, and/or the education of the consumers of medical care. This will necessarily have to be a largely theoretical task, not because there is no evidence, but because the evidence goes in the same direction. What evidence there is suggests that CME of professionals makes little if any difference in their subsequent performance. And the evidence about the impact of consumer education is about the same: there is little solid evidence that individuals significantly alter their behavior on the basis of information about their health.

Happily, both of these assertions need some qualification.

The Evidence About CME for Professionals

If it is said that continuing education does not work, what does that mean? Stripped down, what it appears to mean is that programs designed to refresh a professional's skills have not been shown positively to alter subsequent performance on the job. This does not mean that such programs cannot work; it just means that there is not much reliable evidence that they do.

There could be many reasons for this sorry state of affairs. First, the measures that have been used to assess subsequent performance might not have been sensitive enough to capture modifications in practitioner behavior. Second, the program content of continuing education might not have been sufficiently related to on-the-job performance — not too surprising, since professional education itself is rarely related. And third, it could be that professionals do not take the programs seriously enough.

Yet it remains troubling that we cannot conjure up some success stories because CME is such a piquant idea — such a nice, cheap, and easy way to combat professional blundering. And too, there are some benefits to the programs which perhaps cannot (or at least should not) be measured. What's wrong with a little professional R&R; a little collegiality and gin shared across sputtering golf carts? CME programs can undoubtedly be improved by aiming them toward specific instances of provider incompetence. Armed with PSRO revelations, CME programs could become a reasonably potent tool to reeducate individual miscreants, even if, in the aggregate, the evidence remains indifferent.

In sum, though the research record is not promising, the market for continuing education couldn't be better. Everyone is for it, principally because it will buy some more precious time and insulation from the federal government, who some say would otherwise climb all over the doctors about their performance. And there is, even at the same time, some hope that CME could be made to work a little bit better.

Of course, there is more to it. There are at least three more reasons why it hasn't worked. The first is the simplest: people really have not been serious enough about CME to make it work. Professionals are not uneducable, but long-ingrained patterns of behavior cannot be changed by weekend conferences alone.

Second, and related to the first, changes in professional behavior can probably be achieved if program content is squarely focused on the practice shortcomings of individual providers based on hard evidence (evidence which should soon be available from PSRO programs)—*and* if appropriate but effective behavioral rewards are introduced. If a practitioner can be shown that better performance is cost-effective, he or she might respond more positively; physicians have long shown an alarming capacity to respond to fiscal incentives. A weekend frolicking in Aspen is hardly a "professional obligation" as professional organs sonorously claim; but a weekend program in Toledo, Ohio, in a facility well equipped for learning and not play, coupled with well-tailored follow ups, might have a chance.

The third reason is both more serious and more troubling. There is a myth in the land that the problems of quality in medical care can be blamed on a few less than fresh apples in a barrel teeming with bright red and healthy ones. Based on the evidence there is, this is an unvarnished excuse. True, there are undoubtedly a few real bunglers—physicians who should be gracefully retired to the cribbage boards. But the available research makes it clear that the problems of quality are largely systemic problems—not individual ones.[2] In other words, it's not as if some apples are rotten and others are fresh; the barrel itself seems to be falling apart. Patients do not usually get mangled by individuals (although once in a while that happens); patients do get mangled by systemic faults that make perfection impossible. Satisfactory performance at best seems an attainable but difficult goal.

Unless these considerations are discussed openly, CME will continue to be peripheral to good medical care, however central it may be to the psycho-social needs of the practitioner.

Now for the other shoe.

The Evidence About Consumer Health Education

It would be a matter of great glee for me to unequivocally state that consumers have been shown to respond to health education programs. But the evidence just is not there. No matter that their failure to respond might be the result of decades of being told they were stupid; a positive self-image and a reasonable degree of confidence are essential prerequisites for behavioral change. But patients have usually been told to shut up and submit. But even if tomorrow all patients were told that they were smart, and they believed it, it would take many years to achieve results — people do not suddenly become smart.

And to top it off, we consumers *really* are dumb — without a doubt. Dumb is not being able to pump up an armband and read the silly little gauge. Dumb is not being able to read a chart. Dumb is not insisting on being told just a few simple things, such as what the alternatives are to surgery or what the alternatives might be to heavy doses of strange multicolored pills. Dumb is not knowing that lumps in the breast are not migrating marbles. And finally, Dumb is not recognizing the simple relationship between what one sticks in one's mouth, how often, and in what amount, and human health.

This, then, is a serious problem. Not only have we been told that we are dumb, but we are dumb! No wonder health education is a problematic affair — it is trying to teach retardates how to build jet engines. We have a long way to go. Perhaps the first step is to stop telling people that they are dumb; to begin to trust them with some information and with some tools for their own care. Although this will not do it alone; consumer education will take time.

But, bear in mind how resoundingly dangerous such a step would be. The very foundations of medicine would begin to shake. Patients could become participants in their own sickness and producers of their own health — an anathema.

But there is no cause for great worry; the odds are not too great. Health education, it is said, does not work.

ANOTHER LOOK AT THE EVIDENCE

As noted, existing evidence there is bleak. Consumers have shown that they can effectively participate as managers of medical care facilities and programs, although they rarely challenge the professional on matters of clinical competence. But when one considers measurable behavioral change in response to information about their health — the research results are not promising. But given the dogged hopes and aspirations of health education advocates, we should look harder.

The persistence of smoking in the face of incontrovertible evidence about its danger to human health is usually cited as the major evidence of the consumer's failure to respond. And it is true that the data show only a slight slowing in the rate of increase in smoking since the surgeon general's belated warnings on the subject. But this finding has to be taken apart.

What the evidence does show is that certain population cohorts have responded to the exhortation. Physicians, young married men (particularly those with children), and pregnant women have all significantly responded to the stimulus. Unfortunately, these gains have been almost entirely offset by an increase in the rate of smoking among young teenage women. So even though the gross results are not necessarily promising, further examination of the responses of particular population cohorts gives us something to go on. For example, the data suggest that people who have some reason to be concerned about their health and are not necessarily vulnerable to psycho-social pressures to smoke do indeed respond. Moreover, the inference can at least be drawn that when those psycho-social inducements which bear so heavily on young teenage women wane, as they grow older, they, too, will perhaps alter their behavior.

But, there is even more evidence. When it began to be reported in the press that eggs might be harmful because of their contribution to cholesterol levels in the blood, the consumption of eggs dropped dramatically. No research was trumpeted to prove this. But there were alarms sounded by egg producers and food producers relying on egg products. Hence, in the real world market of egg yolks, bacon and eggs, greasy breakfasts, and omelets, consumers really responded to scattered information about the potential dangers of the bounty of chickens.

Another source of "proxy" information is the boom in sales of recreational equipment. Now, it may be true that people are buying tennis shoes, tennis rackets, and running shoes in record amounts and simply carrying them around for show. But if the assumption is made that at least some of them are actually using the stuff, the dramatic increases in the sale of such goods suggests a heightened interest in recreation and exercise.

The last bit of information comes from more rigorous sources. A study commenced in 1972 by Dr. John Farquar and others at Stanford Medical School was designed to test whether consumers would respond to a barrage of information about life style variables and their relationship to heart disease.[3] Three communities in central California were chosen. Each community was about the same size and matched for sociodemographic characteristics. In the first community both printed and visual media were used, together with personal interviews and contacts wherever appropriate and possible. In the second community only printed and visual media were used. A third community served as the control.

The recently reported interim findings show some promise. In the community that was saturated with both visual and printed material (which also benefited from some personal contacts and interviews), behaviors relating to the incidence of heart disease appear to have changed. Overall mortality and morbidity data are significant. In the second community—the community in which only printed and visual media were used—the results were also positive, but not nearly so significant. In the third community things remained about the same.

The final results have yet to be reported (the study is continuing); but the interim results are promising even though, given the costs of the information-dissemination programs utilized in the first community, it can hardly be said that health education has been shown to be cost-effective. So there is some evidence after all, even though it is far from conclusive.

But other factors are also present. I cannot remember my social security number, but I can remember almost any phone number I have used more than two or three times in the last two or three years. Moreover, I can remember almost all book titles, but not very many song titles. You may properly ask why my memory quirks are of any pertinence here. The point is more general. People become smarter if they have a reason to do so. Someone who has never changed a tire will quickly develop the skill if he blows one out on a lonely backroad at three in the morning with a howling wind whipping around him. Until people *want* to learn more about their health, they are not likely to learn very much. The first step toward an effective health education program for consumers is to convince the public that knowing something *can* make a difference. Many people have made significant life style changes after a close brush with death or a severe illness. The trick is to show people that their lives can and will be different if they take charge. Of course this is not easy, but the means must be found to create experiences for people that will give them a sense, an experience, of differences. And since most people visit a doctor or hospital with some frequency, part of the burden to create such experiences might appropriately fall on the professional. This is not to say that doctors should take steps that would harm health to convince patients that death is a real and palpable possibility. But it is to say that health professionals can strenuously remonstrate with patients that the responsibility to be well is theirs. Further, doctors can give their patients some simple guidance and tools about how to take over.

There is another important point. As long as the technology of health education remains at the level of pablum, it will not make any difference whether the teaching techniques are sophisticated or outmoded. We need to be more hard-hitting and relatively fearless. People must be convinced that is is okay to know something about the blood and guts that they walk around in. Rarely does that happen in health education.

Beyond this, as in the case of CME for health professionals, we know enough now about what makes people learn to be a bit more skillful about the techniques that might be used. Consumers will respond to incentives just as doctors do. Not only do we have to find ways to "experience" feeling better, but we must also create incentives for persons to try those methods. Why not reduce health insurance premiums for those who make fewer demands for services; why not reduce benefits for those whose reckless disregard for their well-being results in repeated accidents or illnesses; why not require employers to make recreational and exercise time available to all employees, not just broad-bottomed executives; and why not reimburse providers for health education services?

No miracles can be promised. Health education has never been easy, and is not likely to be any easier in the future. People are refractory critters. No one wants a health czar issuing edicts about the healthy life. Education and incentives seem promising—but ultimately people should have the right to go to the grave clutching their favorite forbidden fruit in each hand. Autonomy probably remains a higher good than health. So be it. But nonetheless, it does seem as if health education is an idea that really has not been tried. It should be.

CONCLUSIONS

My final points are four:

1. Continuing education for health professionals, *unless* radically changed, should be seen for what it is: a fad chasing a whim, both escaping more governmental regulation.
2. Health education for consumers is no panacea and could in fact turn out to be a hollow promise. Just because it has not been tried does not mean that trying it will make it work. But, given the costs of care and the walls we have run into in all directions of trying to work ourselves through the crises of modern medicine, it seems worth trying.
3. Consumer education could turn out to be the most effective form of CME for professionals. Not only will well-informed and aware consumers make fewer unnecessary demands on physicians and hospitals, but also the possibility for increased health professional awareness is equally great. Consumers who are not uninformed, who really communicate and participate in their care and in taking care of themselves, will have a lot to teach the doctor about how human organisms function in states other than those abject and paralytic states in which many now present themselves for medical care. Indeed, why not organize health education programs in which health professionals and consumers participate as both listeners and presentees—think about that for a moment.
4. My last point is similar to my first—consumer health education must be seen for what it is—the beginning of the end of professional dominance (if it works). Eliot Freidson will not have any more books to write; and if that isn't tragedy enough, people might start taking care of themselves and stop going to doctors so much. And then society will have even more unused hospital beds. Doctors will have time to play more golf or tennis. Of course, we could always use some hospitals for arts and crafts shows, and then, too, we could possibly retrain some doctors to be investment counselors.

NOTES

1. I owe the germ of this idea to Al Jonsen at the Health Policy Program at the University of California Medical School in San Francisco.

2. See, in particular, Robert Brook, *The Halothane Study* and the more recent "institutional differences" study conducted by researchers at Stanford University.

3. For a report on the study, see Charlotte K. Byers, "Can Health Habits Really be Changed?" *Prism* 2 (May 1974): 13-17.

Part VI
Issues for Policy Consideration

Chapter 20
Policy Issues and Conclusions

Staff of the Boston University Health Project

(The statements printed below in bold face, excerpted from the proceedings of the study conference, are representative of the major viewpoints expressed.)

In recent years almost half the states in the nation have passed laws that require physicians to participate in a stipulated number of hours of formal CME "course-work," as a condition for maintaining their license to practice medicine; additional states are now actively considering similar action. In large part this trend results from a virtual explosion of professional, consumer and government interest in efforts directed at quality assurance in medicine; and, particularly in the last two years, it also represents a byproduct of the malpractice crisis.

> **The public simply demands that something be done to ensure them that their physicians are competent to practice medicine. And since we really don't know what that something is, the only thing we have is education. It seems to be the most harmless method to assure that physicians are competent, and the public seems to be in general agreement that this is somehow effective. So education has filled the vacuum.** *George J. Annas*

Although voluntary CME has been present and expanding each year for the past half century in the United States, mandatory CME is qualitatively and quantitatively a new issue. The views of the medical community, both practitioners and educators, range from solid support of the mandatory trend and belief in its effectiveness to improve the quality of care, to warnings of great danger to the free practice of medicine. Some of the extreme views can be written off as the "blind enthusiasm" of a few; but there is serious division about the wisdom and effectiveness of the current CME policy direction throughout the medical community, at both the grassroots and leadership levels.

Many contributors to this volume have serious reservations about the mandatory trend. Some of these reflect doubts about whether most quality problems lend themselves to solution by CME; some stem from concerns over the resource and dollar cost-effectiveness; others result from criticisms about the "form" as opposed to "substance" approach of the requirements; and finally, many reservations relate to doubts about the technical and logistical feasibility of adequately evaluating the impact of CME programs and requirements.

> I guess I agree that, in one sense, requiring mandatory CME hours is harmless because everybody is going to chalk them up anyway. But, in another sense, it is quite disturbing because of the false public expectations that are created when mandatory CME programs are put in place—expectations that in no way are going to be met and that may soon discredit CME altogether. It seems to me that what we need is to take a more aggressive stance. *Michael J. Goran*

Yet, despite the various participants' criticisms and an occasional sentiment that states never should have intruded into the area of CME requirements, no one is about to lead a crusade for repeal, and few appear ready to campaign actively against passage of similar laws in the remaining states.

> Perhaps the time has come to address the question very directly, not expecting to have some magical solution found either in a record system, an audit system, or a formal continuing education system, but really developing a plan for a decade or a generation which has as its goal modifying behavior in the delivery of health care. The time certainly has come to do something different. But it seems to me very unlikely that you are going to do something fundamentally different if we simply try to find the magic bullet that will kill all the enemies that we face. *George E. Miller*

The following sections attempt to summarize and synthesize the perceptions of the Boston University Health Policy Institute staff and our perceptions of the conferees' views, focusing first on the reservations about the effectiveness of mandatory CME and then on the directions for action. Presented here is the Institute's own recommendations for policy makers on the topic of CME and quality assurance.

THE ROLE OF CME IN QUALITY ASSURANCE

Much of the heightened interest in CME is a byproduct of a heightened interest in the quality of medical care delivery. To understand the role of CME in quality assurance, it is necessary, first, to define what CME is supposed to do; second, to delineate the problems of quality care in a framework that is relevant to CME; and third, to project the potential intersection for the application of CME toward achieving quality assurance.

> We have not defined what the limits of continuing medical education are. Is it supposed to correct all demonstrated deficiencies? While it is important to address all kinds of deficiencies, such as deficits in biomedical knowledge as well as comunication skills, interview skills, time management, personnel management, etc., I think it is unrealistic to attempt to address certain problems over which one has no control, such as the deficits produced by a hostile physician. *Leonard Rubin*

CME is a generic term for a loosely grouped collection of activities whose broad spectrum includes the use by an individual physician of journals and/or tape cassettes; didactic lectures before large audiences at professional meetings; self-assessment examinations offered by specialty societies; "tailor-made" programs of instruction designed by medical schools; local hospital staff conferences and rounds; and numerous other variants. By definition, the audience is physicians who have completed their undergraduate (medical school) and postgraduate (internship, residency, and specialty fellowship) training, and who, for the rest of their professional careers, will be partaking of "continuing" education.

> The farther you go in the circle beyond the level of immediate knowledge and competence of the individual, the more difficult it is to prescribe through the nature of the educational process that your efforts will result in improved patient care. There are lots of reasons why people do what they do, and what they know is only one of them. I think that maybe we ask too much of continuing medical education in that sense. *C. H. William Ruhe*

The central and short range technical objectives of most CME efforts are to transmit new information (primarily new knowledge and, to a lesser degree, new skills) and/or to refresh or restimulate old knowledge and skills, building on a core of knowledge and skills developed during undergraduate and postgraduate medical education. The longer range objectives of CME efforts (usually not well defined) also vary markedly and may include diffusion of new diagnostic and therapeutic modalities into clinical practice, enhancement of the "quality" with which current modalities are applied, simple acquisition of knowledge for the sake of individual intellectual satisfaction, and combinations of these and other objectives. The motives for participation by physicians can range from the altruistic (such as wanting to be able to offer the newest and best care to patients) and the pecuniary (such as learning a new office procedure that Blue Shield will reimburse at $50 per application) to the sustenance of one's livelihood (i.e., license) because of mandatory state CME requirements.

The most serious—and most publicized—problem in quality assurance is that there is a small but very real group of physicians who, as individuals, consistently practice poor quality medical care; this group is often referred to as "the bottom five percent" or the "black hats" of the medical profession. Upon closer examination, this group consists of three types of physicians:

1. physicians who have serious personal problems, such as drug addiction, alcoholism, physical/mental disabilities, or psychiatric disorders, that affect their practice performance;

2. physicians who repeatedly perform unwarranted procedures and schedule unnecessary visits or tests for their patients; and

3. physicians who have become so sloppy about their maintenance of skills and knowledge that over a period of years, as the standard of practice changes due to new knowledge of diagnosis and treatment, they become increasingly out of step with what is considered adequate medical skills.

In looking at CME and the PSRO role, we have to think in terms of the whole population of physicians, not a subpopulation of 'outlyers' or 'black hats.' This subpopulation of really inadequate providers may be dealt with by PSRO-type educational techniques. But traditional CME will for the foreseeable future still have the primary responsibility of moving the entire population of practitioners toward better performance.
Alan R. Nelson

It is difficult to believe that the first two types of physicians, and the quality problems they represent, will be affected by any type of CME program. Those individuals must be detected and dealt with by PSROs, medical society grievance committees, hospital privilege committees, and state licensing boards. It is only the third type of "deficient" physician who would benefit from CME and whom the public would have reason to force to participate. The number of physicians in this third subgroup probably represents only a small fraction of what is at its largest probably a small total group. Though no one has any hard data, the third type probably represents only one percent of practicing physicians.

For the remaining vast majority of physicians, who—on an average—practice at an acceptable quality of care, there are two different dimensions of quality that have become of concern. One is the technical, scientific quality of their practice, and the other is the nontechnical or "art of caring" aspect. Although the principal emphasis in medical education has been given to the more scientific aspects of medical practice, in recent years there has been increasing concern within the medical education leadership about deficits in the "caring" aspects of practice. However, many feel that humanism in practice is not a new area of knowledge that develops after a doctor graduates from medical school, or a knowledge or skill that can deteriorate, but instead represents a set of interpersonal skills in which the physician has received insufficient training during his undergraduate and postgraduate education. Thus, there is little for CME programs to build on or refresh. The quality problems in "caring" require reform in the medical schools, not new types of, or requirements for, CME.

> When people get out to medical school and we find that they are not independent learners, we complain about them rather than about ourselves, who have fostered and rewarded such an educational goal. We ought to devote far more attention to this problem at the undergraduate and graduate level than we have done. *George E. Miller*

The quality aspects of "good" doctors, in the technical areas of medical practice, can usually be classified as one or both of the following types:

1. failure to *possess* appropriate information considered necessary to meet quality standards; and/or
2. failure to *apply* such information.

The former type could result from inadequate information received in medical school, forgetting information previously learned, new diagnostic and therapeutic information arising after formal training, or receiving inappropriate information (e.g., misrepresentations by drug salesmen). The latter problem can be due to sloppiness, failures in judgment, and other factors inherent to the physician and/or related to external pressures (e.g., twenty patients who must be seen in an hour).

> **It is dangerous to try to evaluate the continuing education experiences of physicians by looking at the quality of care. There are just too many variables that have a bearing on health care quality.** *Robert A. Chase*

In theory, CME should serve as a principal device for solving the problems of physicians not possessing adequate information. However, participants at the conference and other experts who have studied quality-of-care problems believe that:

1. In quantitative terms, failures to *apply* knowledge of good medical practice are vastly more significant than failures to *possess* knowledge; and
2. Except for lack of knowledge about new developments, the quality problems related to knowledge deficit often do not show consistent patterns (e.g., in a group of 100 physicians it is more likely that there will be 100 different deficits than that there will be a single common deficit)—a fact that makes it difficult, and often costly, to develop an effective continuing education program.

> **The key question is how often lack of information or knowledge is the problem in poor quality of care. Almost invariably, the physician knows about five times as much as what he's doing— so the problem isn't lack of knowledge. And yet we treat the poor quality of care almost always as though it were a lack of knowledge.** *Clement R. Brown, Jr.*

These beliefs were expressed most strongly by critics with experience in the PSRO program. They also felt there was a similar problem with patterns of specific single instances of failure to apply knowledge. When consistent patterns of either type were found, they felt that standard CME techniques of lectures at professional meetings, hospital conferences, written materials, etc., could be very effective in improving the quality of medical care. However, quality problems that are random across groups of physicians or consistent only within the practice of a random individual physician could probably be dealt with most effectively by the use of individualized warnings and sanctions (the "tap on the shoulder" by the peer review committee) and the development of individualized programs of CME (for instance, self-assessment exams).

> We've come to the point in PSRO development where we're really going to test the willingness and the ability of the medical profession and practitioners participating in PSRO to use PSROs as change agents to improve performance. The tools are there and have been adequately demonstrated to be capable of assessing deficiencies in performance. The problem still is how to actually achieve change. PSROs have the authority to do this, with their payment and sanction authorities. But there is yet no clear indication that there is willingness to apply them in a way way to actually produce change. *Michael J. Goran*

> We have been successful in changing the behavior of physicians. The improvements we have found rarely result from a formal educational activity such as a lecture. Improvements follow such activities as a one-on-one discussion with a physician or an announcement of the audit results in the hospital newspaper. *Leonard Rubin*

FORM, COSTS, AND EVALUATIONS OF MANDATORY CME

Much of the criticism of CME is directed not at all types of CME but toward the requirements associated with manditory CME. The following are some of the major criticisms:

First, CME requirements usually are characterized by fixing a number of formal course hours of accredited CME to be taken each year, but they give very limited credit for any self- instructional CME time (e.g., reading journals or using audio cassettes) or informal group instruction (attending grand rounds at the university medical center, participating in hospital staff conferences). The latter methods can be equally, if not more, effective than formal lectures or seminar sessions given by an accredited CME program.

Second, there are no stipulations that the CME course work has any relevance to the physician's practice. For example, a pediatrician could take forty hours of CME courses in neurosurgery each year, thus fulfilling the requirements for maintaining his license. How his young patients would benefit from this is hard to understand. Further, since there are no required exams or questions of attendees, credit is received for simply being present, not for proof of learning.

> We should develop mechanisms of providing information that are built into the health care system at a time when the information is needed, that is, at the time the problem list, the diagnostic plan, and the therapeutic plan are being evolved. Computer technology makes this accessing and displaying of the information possible. Efforts in this direction are more significant than aimless discussion that beats the lecture to death by saying it can't teach. It certainly can teach, but it teaches at the wrong time, before the information is needed, rather than at the time it is needed.   *Philip R. Manning*

Third, there is little evidence to support the contention that formal CME course work either increases a physician's knowledge base or, more important, improves his performance (i.e., the quality of care delivered to patients). In fact, except for a few noteworthy cases, there has been almost no rigorous evaluation of the structure, techniques, or results or CME programs. The "outcome" of CME has probably been one of the most underfunded areas of research by the Department of Health, Education, and Welfare.

> You may not be able to demonstrate any change as a result of having done [CME], but if you didn't do it there certainly would be a change over a period of time—a change for the worse.
> *C. H. William Ruhe*

> There are reasonably solid evaluation studies available which have indicated (a) that traditional CME is not very effective in improving performance in the health-care-delivery system, and (b) that the audit method can in fact identify deficiencies through its assessment mechanisms that can be individualized, and that these deficiencies can be corrected if the institution or the individuals involved make the appropriate changes and carry out the changes that are required.   *Michael J. Goran*

Fourth, there is little quality control or monitoring of the teachers and organizers of CME programs. Once a program, such as a Department of Continuing Education at a medical school, has been accredited, the quality of the instruction in its CME courses is generally not examined in depth. Often the standards of evaluation are the number of physicians who attended and the amount of profit made on the CME program.

> The only excuse for teaching is to help someone learn something, and learning is defined as a change in behavior, not as exposure to something that you are taught. Thus, if we don't change behavior, then we are failing in our mission; and, as good scientists, we ought to look systematically and objectively at what we are doing. We must be sure that this enormous investment of billions of dollars is invested in something that has a higher probability of payoff than the kinds of things we are engaged in now. *George E. Miller*

Fifth, many supporters as well as critics are concerned about the resource and dollar costs to society of mandatory CME. Even a minimal requirement of 10 hours of course work annually for all physicians in the United States would consume approximately three million hours of physician time. Though not all of this would represent time taken from patient care, if only one-third were diverted from service (the other two-thirds from physicians' current educational and leisure time), this would represent a potential loss of approximately six million patient care visits. At what point to the purported health benefits to patients of "better-educated" physicians become negative in relation to the benefits that might be obtained from more patient care by "lesser-educated" physicians? There are two additional costs: first, the time that CME faculty might have spent training new health professionals; second, the loss of tax revenues to the federal government (and some state governments) from tax deductions for CME.

There are many who believe that appropriately designed mandatory CME efforts may be both cost-and quality-effective but doubt that a "shotgun" approach of mandating an arbitrary number of CME hours will meet those objectives.

> One of my concerns is that by requiring hours of traditional continuing education for relicensure or recertification, the profession and the licensing boards and specialty organizations may

feel that they have discharged their responsibility, and we may be lulled into a false sense of security about the needs that exist for assuring quality. *John A. D. Cooper*

THE FUTURE OF CME

Most critics contend that it would be futile to try to turn the clock back on the trend toward nationwide mandatory CME. There is a sense that state governments want to take some visible action in the area of improving the quality of physician performance, that criticism of mandatory CME is often regarded as a simple defensive reaction by the medical profession, and that, until proven substitutes can be offered, the profession is going to have to live with mandatory CME.

I think it would be ill-advised at this stage to link any form of mandatory or pressure-oriented education with PSRO, which would act to strengthen that regulatory arm. I think instead you really ought to act to strengthen the alternatives to regulation. The medical audit is on a more voluntary basis, and I think this should be strengthened. *Edward Roberts*

Given the force of mandatory CME, how do you put rigor into the system that is going to be there? How do you try to ensure that those experiences have an optimal chance to be of value? To me, that's the issue. The issue is not how to stop it. *William D. Mayer*

Further, many speakers felt that while policy makers should continue to be cautioned about the lack of potential of CME for solving the malpractice and "black hat" problem, the profession should now try to harness these requirements, develop modifications, and take other constructive actions to improve CME in ways that would benefit both physicians and patients in the most cost-effective manner. In supporting this view, one participant at a CME conference said:

The time has come when we must acknowledge that social forces are leading to some kind of requirement for, not participation in medical courses, but for assurance of continuing competence of practitioners. It is not realistic to call for a moratorium. It is both realistic and a positive contribution to point out that what we have done in the past seems to be limited in its vision of what continuing education is, and limited in its impact upon professional competence. But we should move forward to use the present opportunity that society seems to be presenting us to improve this process.

Part VII

Policy Recommendations of the Boston University Health Policy Center

Chapter 21
Policy Recommendations

Many states are either moving toward or have already instituted requirements for mandatory participation in continuing medical education programs. **Rather than attempting to halt this movement, a concerted effort should be made to build on the interest and concern these requirements generate and use this opportunity to improve the way CME is currently carried out.** To accomplish this, the following specific steps are recommended. Since responsibility for their implementation must be shared by all the major parties involved in CME activities, particular attention is given to identifying the specific actions that each of these groups must take in working together to improve the process of continuing medical education.

1. A clear distinction should be made between (1) assuring the public of minimum standards of acceptable physician performance, and (2) assuring the delivery of high quality medical services. Although both goals are important and should be pursued, a distinction between the two is necessary if the mechanisms developed to achieve them are to be effective.

- **Minimum standards for licensed M.D.s.** *State licensing bodies* have primary responsibility for assuring minimum levels of competency and performance. Mandatory CME will be used by some boards to assist them in fulfilling this responsibility. State boards also have the responsibility of disciplining incompetent and errant practitioners.
- **Continued competence and quality of care.** *Medical schools and physician organizations* will continue to be the primary resource for sponsoring and implementing CME programs. In the current furor over mandatory CME, their principal goals should be:
  a. to provide support and assistance to the many state and local

237

groups who will need help in carrying out mandated programs, and

b. to continue (and expand) their current efforts to develop mechanisms for assuring both continued physician competence and high quality care delivery. Alternative approaches should continue to be tested in developing these assessment mechanisms, and particularly in attempting to develop meaningful procedures for recertification requirements, specialty societies should give careful attention to ensuring that assessments are based not only on physician knowledge but also on a wide range of performance skills as well (including those relating to patient management and education).

2. **Particular effort must be made to maximize the potential of the Professional Standards Review Organization mechanism as an educational vehicle.** The federal government must plan and implement its regulatory, administrative, and funding actions to assist private and public groups at the state level that are working to improve CME efforts. Problems in care delivery identified through the quality assurance and peer review activities of PSROs, and the data that they will have on such problems, can be a vital resource in both planning and evaluating CME programs. In addition to the federal initiatives required, both the *medical schools and private medical organizations* should attempt to work out cooperative programs with the PSROs in their areas. Initial cooperative steps require very little investments and need not wait until actions such as federal funding PSRO educational activities take place.

3. Special attention should be given to **broadening the scope of CME activities.** In particular, careful consideration should be given to allowing requirements for physicians (whether established on a voluntary or mandatory basis) to be met through a variety of CME approaches, and these should not be limited solely to the traditional lecture/course format. Some redirection in current and future investments in CME is needed to enable the parallel development of such alternative approaches as **performance-based programs** and others focused on patient management and communication skills and patient involvement in the educational process. Each of the major participants in CME activities must contribute to this effort to expand and improve the continuing education process:

- *State governments* that have passed mandatory CME requirements should provide "seed" money to stimulate both the development and evaluation of alternative CME approaches and should also encourage the development of private support for such studies. Documentation of the costs and benefits of different strategies is needed to guide policy development, both in those states that already have mandatory requirements and in those where a decision on the question has not yet been made (thus enabling comparisons and assessments of the impact of mandatory requirements).

- The *federal government* should undertake a major program of research, development, testing, and evaluation of CME approaches and the impacts that these approaches have on physician skills and patient results. No private or public organization at the state level has the resources to undertake such efforts; moreover, many of the important evaluations involve comparisons of programs *between* states. Unless the federal government undertakes such actions, there will be little capability to improve CME and an increased probability that physician time and tax subsidies (in the form of physician tax deductions for CME expenditures) will be spent on an activity that is unproductive in terms of improving the health of the public.

4. Recognition must be made that education to improve patient care encompasses all levels of medical training and is a process in which practitioners participate throughout their careers. To be effective, the continuing education process must be a fundamental part of the early learning experiences of medical students. As further effort is made to relate CME strategies more directly to performance in care delivery, *medical schools* must carefully evaluate the degree to which quality-of-care problems, both in a technical as well as an "art of caring" sense, are due to deficiencies in medical student and house staff training rather than to gaps in the knowledge gained through continuing education. Much greater emphasis in the learning process should be placed on patient management and communication skills and on methods of assessing performance.

5. In attempting to move toward national and regional coordination in the development, implementation, and evaluation of CME activities, actions are needed first at the state level, as recommended above, to attempt to integrate CME-related activities of government agencies with those in the private sector. Rather than deciding now whether national coordination is appropriate and feasible and, if so, who should be given overall responsibility for accomplishing it, the first priority must be to develop better regional cooperation and to improve the operation of CME through the avenues suggested here.

Index

A

Accreditation, of institutions, 7
Adverse drug reactions, 199—204
Alcohol, Drug Abuse, and Mental Health
  Administration, 150
American Academy of Family Practice,
  148, 152
American Academy of General Practice,
  63, 64, 68
American Academy of Medical Colleges,
  177, 191, 192
American Board of Allergy and
  Immunology, 53
American Board of Colon and Rectal
  Surgery, 53
American Board of Family Practice
  (ABFP), 51
  and CME, 63—65, 68, 148
  and mandatory recertification, 63—65,
  68, 153
American Board of Internal Medicine, 52,
  72, 175
American Board of Medical Specialties
  (ABMS)
  certification, 51
  examination, 41
  recertification, 52, 56, 61
American Board of Nuclear Medicine, 53
American Board of Ob-Gyn, 53
American Board of Ophthalmology, 53
American Board of Otolaryngology, 53
American Board of Pediatrics, 175

American Board of Physical Medicine
  and Rehabilitation, 53
American Board of Plastic Surgery, 53
American Board of Radiology, 53
American Board of Surgery, 42, 53,
  72, 175
American Board of Thoracic Surgery, 53
American Cancer Association, 148, 203
American College of Physicians, 39, 148
American College of Surgeons, 39, 43, 148
American Diabetes Association, 203
American Heart Association, 148, 203
American Lung Association, 148
American Medical Association (AMA)
  and CME, 3—4, 53, 146, 147, 152,
  169, 190
  House of Delegates and PRA, 3
American Osteopathic Association, 147,
  152

B

Benefit/cost analysis
  benefit potential evaluation, 111, 113,
  115, 152—156
  and CME, 109, 122—123, 124, 152—156,
  238—239
  costs of CME, 120—122, 231
  principles, 110—112
  time evaluation, 11, 114, 122
"Bi-Cycle" model, 11—13, 43, 97
Brown, Clement R., 82, 97
Boston University Health Project, 223—233

Boston University Health Policy Center, 237—239
Bureau of Quality Assurance, 73, 150

C

Center for Disease Control, 150
Certification, 58, 59, 60
  See also Recertification;
  Relicensure
Computers
  role in education, 86, 191—192
Confidentiality
  physician, 40
Consumer education, 195—207, 211-218
Continuing medical education (CME)
  alternatives to, 163—171, 195, 211—218
  ABFP recertification, 63—65
  benefits of programs, 112—117
  "Bi-Cycle" model, 11—13
  costs, 109, 111, 117—119, 143—158, 231
  criticisms, 15, 17, 34—37, 43, 165—168, 174—175, 212—214
  deductibility of expenses, 132—138
  evaluation, 13, 84—85, 94—99, 119—126
  federal government, 69—70, 73, 149—151, 239
  funding, 32, 113 n, 120—122
  general practitioners, 79—80, 82
  health care quality, 6—7, 34, 49, 73, 79, 110, 173—174
  hospital role, 83—85, 145—146, 181, 186—187, 188, 191
  IPP, 19, 22
  IRC, 131—140
  industry role, 148—149
  Kaiser-Permanente, 30
  mandatory participation, 9, 109, 174, 223—224, 229—232
  medical association role, 147
  medical school role, 146—147, 173, 178, 181, 183—189
  medical society role, 147—148, 181, 189—191
  peer review, 37
  physicians, 123, 124, 144—145
  PRA, 3
  professionalization of, 82, 117
  proposals, 168—171, 232—233, 237—239
  proposed national academy, 170
  PSRO role, 101, 104, 106
  public accountability, 72, 164—165
  public policy, 156—158
  recertification, 53, 61, 73
  relicensure, 71, 73
  SESAP, 39—43
  state government, 69—74
  tax law, 131—133, 139
Cooperative education program, 195, 203, 204
Coordinating Council on Medical Education (CCME)
  recertification, 59—60
Cost/benefit analysis
  See Benefit/cost analysis
Croul, Dr. Richard, 149

D

Darley, Ward, 168, 170
deDombal, I.T., 85—89
Department of Defense, 151

E

Escovitz, G.H., 96, 97, 98
Evaluation of education programs
  methodology, 47—56, 61
  validity, 49, 61
Expenses
  deductibility of CME costs, 132—140

F

Federal Drug Administration (FDA), 150
Federal government, 58, 69—70, 73, 149—151, 157, 239
  certification requirement, 58
  CME, 69—70, 73, 149—151, 239
  medical audit, 73
  recertification, 58
  relicensure, 58, 157
Flexner Report, 64
Fox, Dr. E.R.W., 156

H

Health, Education and Welfare (HEW)

Task Force on Prescription Drugs,
198, 199
Health Maintenance Organization (HMO),
164
Health Services Administration, 150
Hill v. Commissioner of Internal Revenue,
134
Hospitals
accreditation requirement, 58
community, teaching, and specialty,
83–85
CME, 83, 84, 85, 145–146, 191

I

Illinois Council on Continuing Medical
Education (ICCME), 147
Individual Physician Profile (IPP)
CME, University of Wisconsin, 19
criticisms, 23
ICDA, 20
patient record, 26
physician deficiencies, 23–26
purpose, 22
study results, 20–22
Insurance carriers, 59, 60, 70
Internal Revenue Code (IRC), 131–140
International Classification of Diseases,
Adapted (ICDA), 20
Internists, 80, 82

J

Joint Committee on Accreditation of
Hospitals (JCAH), 157, 203
certification, 58
CME, 145
recertification, 58

K

Kennedy, President John F., 133
Kennedy, Senator Edward, 58

L

Lee, Dr. Phillip R., 149
Licensure, 50, 65–66, 237
See also Certification

M

McCormack, Dr. J.C., 143
Maloney, James V., Jr., 43
Malpractice, 59, 70
Manpower supply
quality of health care, 90
Medicaid, 69–70
Medical associations
and CME, 147
Medical schools
and CME, 146–147, 177, 181, 183–189
evaluation of health care problems,
239
Medical societies
and CME, 181, 189–191
Medicare, 69–70
Miller, Dr. George E., 152
Morrocco, Dr. John D., 156
Muscular Dystrophy Association, 148

N

National Board of Medical Examiners
(NBME)
physician evaluation, 49, 68
SESAP, 39, 42
National Drug Information Foundation
proposed, 198
National Health Insurance, 90
National Institutes of Health,
149–150
National Library of Medicine, 150
Nelson, Senator Gaylord, 198
Nightingale, Florence, 89
Northern California Kaiser-
Permanente Medical Care Program
and CME, 30, 31, 83
programs, 33

O

Office records
review for recertification, 66
Outcome assessment
IPP, 22–23

P

Patients
    education, 195—207
    noncompliance, 200—204
    records of, 19, 23, 26
    responsibility for quality care,
      11, 13, 14
Peer review
    and quality assurance, 37, 101
    See also Professional Standards
      Review Organization
Peterson, Osler, 152—153
Pharmaceutical industry
    role in education, 149, 204
Phelps, Charles, 114
Physicians
    age factor, 123
    behavior change, 11, 13, 14—15
    CME, 22—23, 123, 144—145
    competency, 72, 237
    Education Program. *See* Continuing
      medical education
    evaluation, 22—23, 26, 176—177
    IPP, 22, 23
    role in patient education, 204
    self-assessment, 20
Physician's Recognition Award (PRA), 60
    AMA costs, 147, 152
    benefits, 113—114
    and CME, 3, 65, 164, 174
    criticisms, 7, 167
    purpose, 3—4
    quality of health care, 5—7
    requirements, 4—5
Problem Oriented Medical Record, 22
Professional Standards Review
    Organization (PSRO)
    CME, 69—70, 150
    education potential, 105, 203, 238
    personnel training, 73
    public accountability, 72, 73, 164
    quality assurance, 102, 157, 175,
      226—229
    relicensure, 73—74
Public accountability
    CME, 164—165
Public policy
    CME investment, 156—158

Q

Quality Assurance Committee
    Kaiser-Permanente, 32
Quality of care
    assurance, defined, 101
    "Bi-Cycle" model, 11—13, 43, 97
    and CME, 49, 79, 95, 97, 110, 124,
      173—174, 225—229
    consumer awareness, 69, 72, 175
    influence of change, 13—16
    Kaiser-Permanente, 29, 34
    licensure, 50
    manpower supply, 90
    organization factors, 83, 85, 98
    patient responsibility, 11, 13, 14
    PRA, 5—7
    recertification, 47—62
    self-assessment methods, 39

R

Recertification
    ABMS, 56—57
    CCME, 60
    CME, 60, 65, 71, 73, 109, 188—189
    costs, 61, 62
    family practice, 63
    JCAH, 58
    malpractice, 59
    mandatory, 52
    quality of care, 47—62
    self-assessment, 60
    specialty boards, 52—53
    specialty societies, 60, 69, 72
    voluntary, 42
Regional Medical Program Service, 163
Relicensure
    CME, 71, 73, 74, 151
    federal government, 58, 157
    PSRO, 73—74
    specialty boards, 69, 72
    state boards, 74
    state government, 58, 157
Richards, Dr. Robert, 50, 53, 157
Rosenow, Edward C., Jr., 39
Rubenstein, Dr. Edward, 154

S

Self-assessment, 53, 60, 67
   See also Surgical Education and
      Self-Assessment Program (SESAP)
Senate health manpower bill, 58
Silverman, Milton, 149
Specialty societies,
   and CME, 148, 190
State government
   certification, 58
   and CME, 69, 74, 149, 238 – 239
   recertification, 58
   relicensure, 58, 157
State societies
   and CME, 109, 147, 190
Steven, Rosemary, 50
Surgical Education and Self-
   Assessment Program (SESAP)
   evaluation, 39 – 43

T

Tax law, 131 – 133
   Tax Reform Act of 1976, 139 – 140

U

University of Nevada College of
   Medical Sciences, 146
University of Wisconsin
   CME, 19, 146
   IPP, 19
Utah Professional Review Organization,
   102
Utilization review, 105

V

Veterans Administration, 151
Voluntary health associations
   CME, 148
   consumer education, 203

W

Welch, Claude, 72
Williams, Senator John, 132
Williamson, John, 82

The Editors

Paul M. Gertman, chief of the Health Care Research Section, Boston University School of Medicine (BUSM), also serves as director of the Health Service Research and Development Program of Boston University Medical Center and director of the Quality Assurance Unit of University Hospital, Boston. He is an assistant professor of medicine and surgery at BUSM. Among Dr. Gertman's principal current research interests are the economic costs to society of various approaches to cancer management; the tradeoffs between preventive and primary-care medicine; and the concept of preventable hospital admissions. He received his A.B. and M.D. degrees from Johns Hopkins University and was a Carnegie-Commonwealth Clinical Scholar there. While on duty with the U.S. Public Health Service, Dr. Gertman was research director of the President's Advisory Council on Management Improvement, a staff member of the Office of Science and Technology, and special assistant to the director of the National Center for Health Services Research and Development.

Richard H. Egdahl is academic vice president for health affairs at Boston University, director of Boston University Medical Center, and executive vice president of University Hospital, Boston. An active surgeon specializing in endocrine surgery, he also directs the Health Policy Institute of Boston University. In the latter role, Dr. Egdahl is director of the Program on Public Policy for Quality Health Care, sponsored by the Robert Wood Johnson Foundation, and coordinates and moderates Administrator's Seminars for the senior staff of the Health Resources Administration of the Department of Health, Education, and Welfare. Among his principal interests in the fields of health planning and health policy are problems of access, cost and quality; manpower and facility distribution; the role of the private sector in financing and organization of primary-care models; and the development of appropriate mechanisms for regulation of the quality of health care. Dr. Egdahl was senior health consultant to the President's Advisory Council on Management Improvement. He studied at Dartmouth College and received his M.D. from Harvard Medical School and his Ph.D. from the University of Minnesota.